Healing the Whole Person

Healing the Whole Person

Integrating Spiritual and Emotional
Care in Clinical Practice

MARY PAMELA EKE

Foreword by Mario Garcia

WIPF & STOCK · Eugene, Oregon

HEALING THE WHOLE PERSON
Integrating Spiritual and Emotional Care in Clinical Practice

Wipf & Stock
An Imprint of Wipf and Stock Publishers
199 W. 8th Ave., Suite 3
Eugene, OR 97401

www.wipfandstock.com

PAPERBACK ISBN: 979-8-3852-6914-3
HARDCOVER ISBN: 979-8-3852-6915-0
EBOOK ISBN: 979-8-3852-6916-7

VERSION NUMBER 01/28/26

Contents

Contents

Illustrations

Foreword

In an era where modern medicine continues to advance through technology and science, Dr. Mary Pamela Eke reminds us that the deepest form of healing begins not in the laboratory but within the human spirit. *Healing the Whole Person* is a timely and transformative work that brings together theology, psychology, and health science to illuminate a truth often overlooked in contemporary healthcare—that wholeness is the harmony of body, mind, and spirit.

As her former professor and dissertation committee chair at Liberty University, I witnessed the birth of this important research and the passion that fueled it. Dr. Eke's study emerged from her ministry as a chaplain serving the diverse community of Swedish Hospital in Chicago, a safety-net institution where cultural diversity, economic challenges, and deep human need converge. Her work responds to a vital question: How can healthcare systems integrate spiritual and emotional care alongside medical treatment to foster holistic healing? Through scholarly rigor, theological reflection and compassionate insight, she identified key themes that shape authentic holistic care, collaboration, communication, support systems, barriers to integration, and the measurable impact of spiritual and emotional interventions. Therefore, it is agreed that when caregivers engage the whole person, addressing fears, beliefs, and meaning as much as physical symptoms, patients experience not only recovery but renewal.

Theologically, Dr. Eke situates her work within a deeply incarnational understanding of healing: Christ's ministry was one of presence, compassion, and restoration. Her framework echoes the words of the apostle John: "Beloved, I pray that you may prosper in all things and be in health, just as your soul prospers" (3 John 1:2 NKJV). In her pages, healing is not merely a clinical outcome but a sacred encounter in which caregivers serve as vessels of divine grace.

This work challenges hospitals, chaplains, and healthcare leaders to reimagine the practice of medicine as ministry, to see each patient as an image-bearer of God, whose suffering deserves not only treatment but tenderness. It calls us to restore what Florence Nightingale called "the spiritual dimension of nursing"[1] and what Scripture names "the balm in Gilead" (Jer 8:22 NKJV).

Dr. Eke's synthesis of pastoral theology and practical intervention creates a model that is replicable, research-based, and infused with faith. It offers a road map for those seeking to embed spiritual care into the culture of healthcare institutions, particularly in times of global uncertainty, burnout, and depersonalization within the caregiving professions. For readers, whether pastors, clinicians, chaplains, or students, this work is both a manual and a meditation. It equips professionals to act, but it also invites them to pause, to listen, to pray, to see the sacred in the suffering. Above all, it rekindles hope that God still heals through the hearts and hands of those who serve.

I commend *Healing the Whole Person* to scholars, practitioners, and faith communities alike. It is a testament not only to Dr. Eke's scholarship and calling but to the enduring truth that when medicine meets ministry, healing becomes whole.

Rev. Dr. Mario Garcia, Esq., DMin, PsyD, DAcHM, MCC
Dissertation Committee Chair
Assistant Professor/Subject Matter Expert (SME)
Licensed Mental Health Counselor & Master Certified Coach (ICF)
Certified Functional & Nutritional Medicine Practitioner
Department of Community Care and Counseling
Liberty University | Training Champions for Christ since 1971

1. Macrae, "Nightingale's Spiritual Philosophy," 8–10.

Acknowledgments

THIS WORK REPRESENTS THE collective efforts, encouragement, and shared vision of my professors, colleagues, and the staff of Swedish Hospital, as well as the unwavering support of my family and friends. Before proceeding further, I wish to express my profound gratitude to God Almighty, whose grace and guidance made it possible for this work to be brought to completion.

To my academic mentors and advisors, especially my dissertation chair, Rev. Dr. Mario Garcia, who also wrote the foreword for this publication, I extend my deep gratitude for your wisdom, guidance, and patience. Your thoughtful feedback strengthened both the rigor and clarity of this work, ensuring that its message remains grounded in both scholarship and practice.

My sincere appreciation goes to the leadership and staff of Swedish Hospital in Chicago, especially my colleagues in Pastoral Care Department and other members of the interdisciplinary team who participated in this study, your openness to this process and your commitment to holistic, patient-centered care provided the foundation for this study. The collaborative spirit I experienced continually reminds me that healing is a shared endeavor, one that thrives through compassion and teamwork.

I also owe a debt of gratitude to my family and friends, whose support and affection kept me going during the long study and writing sessions. I had the strength to finish this project because of your understanding, patience, and steadfast faith in it. You frequently reminded me in subtle ways of the same values this book aims to promote: empathy, human connection, and consideration for the whole person.

I cannot forget to express my deepest gratitude to all of my endorsers. Thank you for your invaluable support, trust, and confidence in my work. Your advocacy has not only validated my efforts, but has also provided the crucial momentum needed to bring this project to fruition. The time and talent you invested into this work cannot be forgotten.

Last but not the least, I would want to thank all medical professionals and spiritual caregivers who commit their lives to helping others. The core of holistic health is embodied in your job, which is frequently invisible and unnoticed. May this book serve as a memento of your devotion and a tool to help you in your on-going work in compassion.

To all who contributed to this journey, in word, in deed, or in spirit, thank you. This work is as much yours as it is mine. I am deeply grateful for the collaboration, mentorship, and inspiration that have sustained me throughout this journey.

Abbreviations

AED	*Automated External Defibrillator*
APC	*Association of Professional Chaplains*
CPR	*Cardiopulmonary Resuscitation*
DMIN	*Doctor of Ministry*
HPCT	*Hospice Palliative Care Team*
IRB	*Institutional Review Board*
NACC	*National Association of Catholic Chaplains*
NIV	*New International Version*
PTSD	*Post-Traumatic Stress Disorder*
RISE	*Resilience in Stressful Events*
SC	*Spiritual Care*

Abstract

IN TODAY'S HEALTHCARE WORLD, we often promise holistic healing, but the results are far less consistent. Although patients receive top-notch medical care, their spiritual and emotional needs are all too frequently neglected. This work fills that gap head-on by providing a way to incorporate emotional and spiritual support into the routine of medical care.

Drawing on qualitative research and insights from interdisciplinary caregivers, this work explores how pastoral care can become a natural part of the healing process rather than an optional add-on. Through thematic analysis, five core ideas emerge: the growing hunger for genuine holistic care, the vital role of support systems, the importance of communication and collaboration among caregivers, the real impact of spiritual and emotional interventions, and the barriers that keep these practices from taking root.

Using a multiple-response coding approach to capture patterns and priorities, the findings point to a simple but powerful truth: when healthcare providers are equipped and encouraged to care for the whole person, body, mind, and spirit, healing becomes richer, deeper, and far more humane.

This book argues that truly holistic care isn't a luxury; it's a necessity. With intentional training and a commitment to seeing patients as full human beings, pastoral and clinical caregivers alike can elevate the healing journey and restore a sense of connection at the very heart of healthcare.

1

Introduction

THE INTERCONNECTED WORLDS OF spiritual care and the practice of holistic healing have arisen as helpful avenues toward a more all-encompassing approach to health and well-being. Regardless of how each person finds or defines their sense of meaning and purpose, all persons need to be cared for physically, spiritually, and emotionally.[1] When one enters any hospital, clinic, or long-term care institution, one can feel it: the hectic bustle, the efforts of medical operations, and the never-ending search for diagnosis, treatment, and repair. It's amazing how modern healthcare can save lives. Despite its sophistication, healing has a more subdued side that is all too often disregarded; this side has nothing to do with technology or medicine but rather with purpose, hope, identity, and connection. Other times, it could be an overwhelming sense of loneliness, guilt, and fear, or ranging from simple spiritual needs, like wanting to feel listened to and valued, to much more complex spiritual needs, like understanding one's place in the world and one's relationship with God and people.[2] Embracing the notion that a person's complete well-being depends not only on the physical body but also on the sustenance of the soul and

1. Kelly et al., *Chaplaincy and the Soul*, 57.
2. Kelly et al., *Chaplaincy and the Soul*, 57.

the cultivation of mental and emotional balance, the combination of spiritual care and holistic healing represents a paradigm shift.

This book was born out of the realization that many patients today are treated with exceptional clinical expertise but without the spiritual and emotional support they need to make sense of their suffering. Even if their bodies have been fixed, their inner lives are still damaged and neglected. In the midst of illness, most patients face questions bigger than their diagnosis: *Who am I now? How do I make sense of this? Where is God in this? What does healing even mean for me?* These are not theoretical questions. They shape how a person experiences illness, copes with fear, and finds the courage to move forward.

However, these spiritual questions are frequently left unanswered, not because patients don't experience them but rather because the clinical environment is not designed to encourage them. Many healthcare professionals feel unprepared to react. A lot of pastoral caregivers and chaplains are overworked. Additionally, a lot of leaders wish to incorporate spiritual care, but many are unsure of how to do so. As a result, the healing process is split, with the physical self getting the majority of care and the emotional, social, and spiritual selves being left on their own.

A rising number of voices from the fields of theology, pastoral care, psychology, chaplaincy, and healthcare have been advocating for an alternative approach during the last ten years. A method of healing that sees individuals as complete beings on a profoundly human journey rather than as symptoms to be treated. A kind of care that acknowledges the spiritual aspect as a necessary companion to the physical, rather than as a supplement. A method that respects the reality that each individual who walks into a hospital bed or examination room has a past, a story, a faith, a fear, a longing, and a hope.

This book is my contribution to that movement. It draws from years of pastoral work, chaplaincy experience, theological reflection, and study with the interdisciplinary team. Based on interactions from the interdisciplinary team, spiritual and emotional care are not peripheral to healing, they are foundational to it. Something changes when patients receive assistance that recognizes their humanity in all its facets. For instance, anxiety becomes less intense, hope comes back, the healing process intensifies, and people find new strength even when they are in pain. But alongside this conviction lies an equally clear reality; most caregivers do not feel equipped or empowered to offer spiritual care. They want to, but they struggle with lack of training, lack of time, and lack of institutional guidance. Many fear crossing boundaries or saying the wrong thing. Others assume that spiritual care belongs exclusively to chaplains. And many chaplains themselves wrestle with workloads that make it difficult to reach every patient who needs them. So, how can we then close this gap between practice and desire? Between what patients require and what caregivers are willing to provide? Between the messy realities of clinical settings and the lovely ideal of holistic healing?

Healing the Whole Person offers a methodology for incorporating spiritual care into professional practice that is accessible, regardless of your role, by combining theological knowledge, practical insight, and research-based understanding. This book is intended to offer you a better understanding of what spiritual care entails, why it is important, and how it can be organically included into daily care, regardless of your role as a chaplain, pastor, ministry leader, doctor, nurse, student, administrator, or community caregiver.

You will hear the voices of caregivers describing what patients truly need. You will encounter themes that emerged repeatedly in this book, the longing for holistic care, the importance of support systems, the power of spiritual and emotional interventions, the challenges of communication, and the barriers that keep spiritual care from flourishing. And you will be introduced to a practical model that helps caregivers see and honor the full humanity of those they serve.

In the end, this book is an invitation to envision a society in which healing is the presence of wholeness rather than just the absence of illness. A future in which hospitals are centers of compassion as well as competence. A society that respects the sanctity of the human experience through therapeutic practice. A world where caregivers from many professions collaborate to address each person's physical, emotional, social, and spiritual needs. Healing the whole person is not a new idea, but it is an urgently needed one. My hope is that this book will give you language, tools, and inspiration to join the movement toward a more compassionate, integrated, spiritually grounded approach to care, one that sees every patient not merely as someone to treat, but as someone to cherish, accompany, and heal.

THE BROKEN LINK IN PATIENT CARE

Despite all the advancements in contemporary medicine that we applaud, there is still a silent fracture at the core of patient care that patients experience profoundly but frequently are unable to identify. It is the feeling that something fundamental is lacking. Despite the fact that healthcare systems are excellent at identifying, treating, stabilizing, and managing illness, many people nonetheless leave their medical visits feeling ignored, invisible, or spiritually lost. The gap between medical care and the deep emotional and spiritual demands that emerge during illness is known as the "broken link."

A person's life can be upended by illness. A diagnosis can cause relationships to fall apart, identity to be disrupted, belief systems to be questioned, and long-suppressed fears to resurface. These difficulties are sometimes more burdensome than the sickness itself, even though patients may not always express them. Even though medical professionals have a great deal of compassion, the system's priorities and speed frequently drive these internal aspects of suffering to the periphery. Accordingly, Roberts asserts, "The spiritual needs of many patients in health care institutions are not being met. All too often, health care workers do not consider the spiritual needs of their patients to be a priority."[3]

Individual clinicians are not to blame for this disparity. It is common for nurses, doctors, chaplains, and other caregivers to say that they would like to provide more comprehensive support but

3. Roberts, *Professional Spiritual and Pastoral Care*, 23.

are limited by time, training, or doubt about how to handle spiritual issues. The healthcare system itself tends to split duties across the interdisciplinary departments. However, patients do not reside in compartments. Their hopes, anxieties, meaning-related queries, and clinical symptoms are all entwined. A vital aspect of healing is neglected when the system isolates the patient's overall experience.

The broken link is not merely the absence of spiritual care; it is the absence of integration. It is the assumption that spiritual and emotional needs can wait until "after the real work is done," or that only certain professionals are permitted to engage these deeper parts of the human experience. This fragmentation leaves patients longing for something more, someone to sit with them through their questions, someone to acknowledge the sacredness of their struggle, someone to see beyond their illness to the person underneath.

It takes more than just suggesting chaplaincy referrals to heal this damaged connection. It demands a change in our conception of healing. Clinicians, chaplains, pastors, and caregivers must all be committed to viewing healing as a holistic process that respects the body without disregarding the spirit. Patients have a greater sense of dignity, purpose, and tranquility when spiritual care is integrated into daily encounters and handled as an essential sign rather than an afterthought.

The broken link can be restored, and when that is done, the experience of care is transformed, not only for patients but for those who accompany them. Caregivers rediscover the meaning of their work, teams communicate more compassionately, and institutions begin to reflect the very humanity they aim to serve. Healing the whole person is not an aspiration; it is a return to what caring has always meant.

MOVING TOWARD INTEGRATED CARE

If the broken link in patient care reveals what is missing, the movement toward integrated care shows us what is possible. Integrated care is not a new invention but a return to a deeply human understanding of healing, one that recognizes the interdependence of body, mind, and spirit. It is the shift from fragmented treatment to relational healing, from isolated tasks to shared purpose, and from a narrow clinical focus to a broad, compassionate vision of the whole person.

Acknowledging that each caregiver has a part to play in meeting patients' spiritual and emotional needs is the first step towards integrated care because one may have a more optimistic attitude toward one's healing process if one feels supported not only in one's physical recovery but also in the person's emotional and spiritual well-being. This does not imply that all clinicians have to become chaplains or spiritual counselors overnight. It entails realizing that, just as important as any prescription or operation, even a brief moment of presence, a kind inquiry, or a sympathetic silence can lead to recovery. Integration is about making connections—between caregivers, between disciplines, and between the patient's internal and external experiences of sickness.

This development necessitates a shift in cultural perspective. Efficiency and clinical accuracy are given top priority in healthcare settings by design. However, integration encourages us to deliberately create environments where chaplains are viewed as partners rather than last-resort referrals, where caregivers are taught to notice indicators of spiritual suffering, and where deeper talks are embraced rather than avoided. In order to provide care that meets patients where they genuinely are, not just physically but also emotionally and spiritually, it encourages teams to interact, exchange ideas, and provide mutual support.

Integrated care also calls for humility and collaboration. The knowledge required to help a patient navigate the complexity of sickness cannot be found in a single discipline. Pastoral leaders carry the larger theological and communal perspective, nurses carry the pulse of the patient's everyday experience, chaplains carry spiritual insight, and doctors carry medical skill. Healing becomes richer, more sensitive, and more compassionate when these voices unite, not in silos but in true partnership.

As we move toward integrated care, we move toward a vision of healthcare where staff feel supported, not overwhelmed; where patients feel accompanied, not managed; and where spiritual care flows naturally within the rhythms of healing. This movement doesn't require massive structural overhauls. It begins with small steps, asking better questions, listening more deeply, collaborating more consistently, and embracing the truth that healing is a shared work.

Thus, integrated care is not merely the future of healthcare; it is the path back to its purpose. It reclaims the age-old knowledge that the best care respects the entirety of the human experience and that people do not heal in fragments. We go closer to healing the whole person and, consequently, reestablishing the core of caregiving itself as we move toward integration.

THE ASSUMPTIONS BENEATH THE HEALING PROCESS

Every approach to care, whether medical, pastoral, or spiritual, is shaped by a set of underlying assumptions. All of them have an impact on how we view patients and address their needs, even though many are not uttered. We are not proposing a method or a favored "style" of care when we discuss treating the whole person. We are relying on a more profound understanding of what it means to be human and to heal. We can operate with clarity, humility, and purpose when we give these presumptions names.

This fundamental idea encourages optimism, resilience, and constructive thoughts by empowering people to take an active role in one's healing process. Assuming that everyone has the capacity for self-healing and growth, spiritual care and holistic healing promote the idea that addressing physical health as well as emotional, mental, and spiritual well-being supports and enhances the body's natural ability to recover, adapt, and thrive. This empowers people to take an active role in one's healing journey and fosters a co-creative environment.

A varied and individual part of the human experience is spirituality. The author holds the assumption that people's feelings of meaning, purpose, and connection to something more than themselves is greatly influenced by one's spirituality. Spiritual care recognizes and encourages one to discover and nurture one's sense of purpose. The underlying premise of "healing and purpose" in spiritual care and holistic healing asserts that people experience higher levels of resilience and well-being when one's quest for wholeness includes not only the restoration of physical health but also the discovery and cultivation of personal meaning. It includes connection to larger contexts, a sense of purpose, and a realization that living in accordance with one's inherent purpose and values plays a crucial role.

Being fully present and mindful is essential for providing spiritual care and facilitating holistic healing. It is a cornerstone of holistic treatment and the provision of spiritual care. It involves cultivating a conscious and non-judgmental awareness of the present moment, both in oneself and when interacting with others. Caregivers can forge sincere relationships, be empathetically sensitive to people's emotional and spiritual needs, and build a safe, compassionate environment for healing by cultivating a strong sense of presence. This process recognizes the interdependence of the mind, body, and spirit, enabling a deeper comprehension of suffering as well as personal development and transformational journeys towards a person's well-being and wholeness.

It is assumed that cultural sensitivity and respect should be demonstrated in spiritual care and holistic therapy. Different spiritual practices and healing philosophies from other cultures should be considered when providing care. Understanding the unique fabric of beliefs, values, and traditions that form people's identities can help people accept and embrace other cultural backgrounds with an open mind and respect. Care providers can personalize one's care to fit the spiritual and emotional needs of each person by appreciating the value of cultural context, creating a climate of inclusivity and trust. According to this viewpoint, cultural understanding not only enhances the healing process but also fosters a closer bond that respects the complexity of human experiences and encourages overall well-being.

A "collaborative approach" stands as a foundational assumption in spiritual care and the realm of holistic healing, emphasizing the importance of a supportive partnership between the caregiver and the care recipient. This approach recognizes that each person holds an innate wisdom about one's own well-being, and the caregiver's role is to facilitate a shared journey of exploration, understanding, and growth. By actively engaging in dialogue, active listening, and mutual respect, caregivers can empower individuals to actively participate in their healing process, fostering a sense of ownership, autonomy, and co-created solutions that integrate physical, emotional, and spiritual dimensions. This approach ultimately underscores that the combined expertise of both the caregiver and the individual serves as a potent catalyst for achieving holistic wellness.

WORDS THAT SHAPE OUR APPROACH

Here, the author looked at necessary definitions of key concepts utilized throughout this book and briefly explained the meanings of these terminologies that are important to the subject. Establishing a common language and context that guarantees readers' understanding of the terms used is vital when the writing digs into difficult subject matter. This section improves the overall clarity, communication, and scholarly rigor of the writing by defining the subtleties and relevance of these concepts, laying the groundwork for a perceptive examination of this writing, and setting the stage for an insightful exploration of the topic at hand.

Cultural competence. Cultural competence involves developing a deep understanding of different cultural norms, values, and practices, and adapting to one's behaviors and communication styles accordingly. According to Lucy and Lavery, "Cultural competence refers to the process of safe delivery of care, which holistically meets the patient's needs, considering cultural aspects."[4] Culturally competent individuals can engage in respectful and meaningful interactions, bridging cultural gaps and promoting inclusivity and mutual understanding.

Cultural sensitivity. "Cultural sensitivity is an essential component of cultural competence and is one of the most important pillars of intercultural communication skills."[5] It involves recognizing and appreciating the diversity that exists among various groups and being mindful of potential cultural differences in communication, behavior, and interactions. Practicing cultural sensitivity fosters inclusivity, minimizes misunderstandings, and promotes effective cross-cultural communication and collaboration.

Emotional care. Emotional care aims to create a safe and nurturing environment where emotions are validated and individuals are empowered to seek the assistance and resources necessary for one's emotional health.

> Emotional care involves providing support and attention to a person's emotional well-being. A better approach to emotional care is the "support response," in which we invite the distressed person to talk more about whatever is bothering them. Allowing someone to talk through their emotions is often the kindest and most supportive thing we can do.[6]

End of life. This phase represents the cessation of functioning, operation, or viability, often marked by a gradual decline or a sudden halt in activity. In the context of living beings, it signifies the natural conclusion of life processes, resulting in death. Nacak and Erden posit that "end-of-life care aims to relieve the pain of the individual in the death process and provide a dignified death experience from the moment when the curative treatment no longer brings any benefit."[7]

---

4. Reeve and Lavery, "Navigating Cultural Competence," 388.
5. Purabdollah et al., "Intercultural Sensitivity," 688.
6. Martelli, *Memory Eternal*, 133.
7. Nacak and Erden, "End-of-Life Care," 142.

Grief. "No matter how many definitions there are to describe grief, the bottom line is this: 'care of those who are grieving is integral to the nature of human beings and deeply present in the spiritual care of those who suffer.'"[8] Garten et al. say that "grief is the normal reaction to a significant loss."[9] It is a complex emotional response to the loss of someone or something significant. Often, it involves a range of feelings such as sadness, longing, anger, and confusion, and can manifest both emotionally and physically.

Holistic care. "Holistic care is a treatment philosophy that sets different and high expectations for standards of care for health care facilities and for all the members of the health care team."[10] This approach seeks to advance general harmony and well-being while acknowledging the interconnection of these dimensions. It entails "determining and meeting the 'spiritual needs' of patients, such as their quest for inner tranquility, the meaning of life, the purpose of suffering, hope, a relationship with God, or 'greater strength.'"[11] It focuses on achieving balance and harmony within these aspects to promote overall well-being.

Interdisciplinary collaboration. Is the "process where individuals from different health professions work together to positively impact patient care."[12] It involves integrating knowledge, methods, and perspectives from multiple academic disciplines to address complex problems or topics. "Through interdisciplinary collaboration, the preferences, hopes, and values of the patient and caregiver can be integrated into the treatment plan, which is key in providing the delivery of optimal care."[13] According to Myrhoj et al., "This collaborative approach integrates the unique skills and expertise of each professional through negotiated interaction, contributing to comprehensive patient care."[14]

---

8. Roberts, *Professional Spiritual and Pastoral Care*, 313.

9. Garten et al., "Palliative Care and Grief Counseling," 6.

10. Roberts, *Professional Spiritual and Pastoral Care*, 22.

11. Klimasinski, "Spiritual Care," 2.

12. Caecilie et al., "Interdisciplinary Collaboration," 2.

13. Caecilie et al., "Interdisciplinary Collaboration," 1.

14. Caecilie et al., "Interdisciplinary Collaboration," 2.

Pastoral care. The care for souls within the Christian religion is referred to as pastoral care and is linked to the notion of guiding. "It represents a means by which the shepherd and leader of the church fulfills his spiritual and social responsibility to the church."[15] "The term 'pastoral' is derived from the Latin term *pascere*, which means 'to feed.' In view of this Latin root, the adjective 'pastoral' suggests the art and skill of feeding or caring for the wellness of others, especially those who need help most."[16] Pastoral care aims to provide shepherding, comfort, guidance, and a sense of connection to one's faith or spirituality during times of need. Thus, "pastoral caregivers who work in secular institutions provide care to religious and nonreligious people alike, and in several Western societies, the term pastoral care is used in relation to nonreligious (humanist) care."[17]

Religious Diversity. According to Lin, "Religious diversity is a social phenomenon in which two or more clearly defined religions exit simultaneously within a region or society."[18] Respecting and recognizing one's freedom to follow one's chosen religion while fostering tolerance, understanding, and peaceful relationships among those from different religious origins is part of the process of embracing religious diversity.

Spirituality. Clyne posits that "spirituality is a broad concept that can include or exclude religion."[19] According to Best et al., "Spirituality is a dynamic and intrinsic aspect of humanity through which individuals seek ultimate meaning, purpose and transcendence, and experience their relationships with family, others, community, society, nature and the significant/sacred."[20] Spirituality is a personal and subjective sense of connection to something greater than oneself. Spiritual beliefs may be religious

---

15. Jibiliza, "Evolution of Pastoral Care," 1.

16. Magezi, "Positioning Care," 2.

17. Schuhmann and Damen, "Representing the Good," 406.

18. Lin et al., "Exploring the Trend," 1.

19. Clyne et al., "Patients' Spirituality Perspectives," e559.

20. Best et al., "Australian Patient Preferences," 1.

or non-religious and can include concepts of the divine, the universe, nature, or inner wisdom.

Spiritual Assessment. Kestenbaum says, "Spiritual assessment is a component of the holistic or biopsychosocial-spiritual approach of caring for the patient."[21] It "enables the chaplain to evaluate the care recipient's spiritual, emotional, and relational resources."[22] Spiritual assessments "summarize and communicate the current spiritual, emotional, and relational state of the recipients of our care."[23] As a dynamic process, "it often begins before we even enter the room with the other."[24] Peng-Keller and Neuhold state that "the purpose of this process is to identify patients/families with potential spiritual or religious struggle, as well as those who would like to receive chaplaincy support."[25]

Spiritual Care. Spiritual care can encompass various practices, including counseling, prayer, meditation, and rituals, tailored to an individual's spiritual beliefs and values. "Our vision of spirituality is closely linked to the ordeal of illness and the suffering it can engender."[26] Spiritual care recognizes the significance of spirituality in a person's overall well-being and aims to promote spiritual growth, understanding, and connection. "When talking about the spiritual dimension of human beings, many works focus on the meaning and ultimate aim of human existence."[27]

Transcendency. Transcendence often goes beyond the experience of ordinary limitations, boundaries, or concepts and is associated with profound spiritual, philosophical, or existential insights. "Self-transcendence is defined as the inner capacity that enables people exposed to stressful life events to find a new purpose and meaning in life."[28] It involves surpassing the usual constraints of

21. Kestenbaum et al., "Spiritual AIM," 415.

22. Peng-Keller and Neuhold, *Charting Spiritual Care*, 34.

23. Peng-Keller and Neuhold, *Charting Spiritual Care*, 33.

24. Peng-Keller and Neuhold, *Charting Spiritual Care*, 33

25. Peng-Keller and Neuhold, *Charting Spiritual Care*, 39.

26. Peng-Keller and Neuhold, *Charting Spiritual Care*, 59.

27. Peng-Keller and Neuhold, *Charting Spiritual Care*, 60.

28. Er et al., "Effect of Psychosocial Distress," 2632.

human perception and understanding, leading to a heightened sense of awareness and connection to something greater than oneself.

Wellness. Wellness is often seen as a dynamic process that involves making positive lifestyle choices and actively pursuing activities and practices that contribute to a state of holistic health. According to Connolly and Oates, "Wellness is not simply the absence of disease. It is a journey of self-awareness to manifest harmony between the various dimensions of well-being in a constantly changing world."[29] It is a state of optimal physical, mental, emotional, and spiritual well-being.

THE FOUNDATIONAL CLAIM

Holistic care of a patient goes beyond the physical illness and its symptoms. This is because, beyond physical health, there lies a web of spiritual and emotional complexities that influence the healing journey. A harmonious healing environment is produced by the interplay of physical, spiritual, and emotional care, which enhances the general well-being of patients. Patients' perspectives on treatment and recovery may be favorably impacted when they feel seen and acknowledged as people with complex needs, not merely as medical cases.

At the heart of this book lies a simple but compelling conviction: healing is most effective, most compassionate, and most transformative when it embraces the whole person, body, mind, and spirit. Every chapter, every example, and every call to reconsider how we treat those who suffer are shaped by this fundamental assertion. It is a claim based on experiences rather than just theory, such as those of patients looking for purpose, caregivers battling burnout, families navigating uncertainty, and chaplains standing by bedsides, where presence becomes the real healing agent instead of words.

The foundational claim insists that spirituality is not an optional add-on or a courtesy extended in moments of crisis.

29. Connolly and Oates, "Wellness Industry," 104.

Instead, it is a core dimension of human experience that shapes how individuals interpret illness, endure hardship, and seek hope. When the spiritual life of a patient is ignored, misunderstood, or dismissed, the care they receive becomes incomplete. Their questions linger unheard, their fears remain unsheltered, and their inner world remains untouched by the healing process.

The idea that the physical body is the primary site of healing and everything else is secondary is another enduring cultural assumption in healthcare that is challenged by this assertion. Even the most cutting-edge treatments cannot completely heal the scars that disease left on identity, purpose, or relationships, despite the remarkable scientific sophistication of modern medicine. People cannot be cured in pieces, but bodies can be treated separately. By addressing the human need for purpose, connection, forgiveness, and direction, needs that become most apparent when life's frailty is exposed, spiritual care fills that gap.

At the same time, the foundational claim affirms that integrating spiritual care is not the exclusive work of chaplains or pastoral caregivers. Instead, it is the shared calling of every person who participates in the healing process. Integration does not require that clinicians become spiritual experts; rather, it invites them to bring curiosity, humility, and presence into their encounters. A nurse's gentle question, a physician's moment of active listening, a social worker's grounding reassurance, each can open a door into the deeper layers of a patient's experience. When chaplains join this collaborative exchange, their expertise enriches the whole system, providing guidance and language for engaging the sacred within suffering.

Ultimately, the foundational claim affirms that holistic healing is not only desirable but essential. It honors the reality that suffering touches every layer of a person's life and therefore requires a response that does the same. It recognizes that caregivers, too, find renewal when they embrace a more integrated model, one that strengthens relationships, deepens purpose, and reshapes the culture of care itself.

2

Conceptual Framework

Understanding what it genuinely means to "heal the whole person" necessitates a thorough understanding of the concepts, practices, and insights that create holistic treatment. This chapter's conceptual framework establishes those guiding pillars, demonstrating how physical, emotional, mental, and spiritual well-being are inextricably linked. By tracing the relationships between these health dimensions, the framework explains why patients' inner lives, beliefs, values, hopes, anxieties, and cultural backgrounds should be central to compassionate care. Rather than addressing sickness as a strictly clinical event, this approach sees recovery as a many-sided human experience.

At the same time, the framework uses known ideas of spiritual care, cultural competency, and whole-person healing to describe how these components interact in practice. It lays the groundwork for understanding the caregiver-patient relationship and how healthcare workers can respond to suffering via presence, empathy, and respect. By laying out the key concepts that guide holistic care, this section prepares the reader to explore the more detailed discussions that follow, including practical models, common challenges, and strategies that help caregivers support genuine healing in every dimension of a person's life.

The theological foundation of this book asserts that human beings are not merely physical entities but also possess an inner dimension that craves purpose, connection, and transcendence. The art of holistic healing, within this theological framework, integrates the dimensions of body, mind, and spirit, acknowledging that true wellness emerges from the harmonious alignment of these angles. With this concept as its theological foundation, spiritual care transforms into a religious undertaking that aims to fulfill the deepest aspirations of the human soul by providing consolation, direction, and solace through times of adversity, pain, and illness.

The idea that the spiritual, emotional, mental, and physical facets of life are inextricably entwined with one another is the theoretical basis for holistic healing and spiritual care. This method recognizes the enormous influence that spiritual ideas, values, and connections have on a person's general health and that true healing goes beyond the relief of physical symptoms. Consequently, the theoretical foundation of this book emphasizes the need to address the spiritual dimension in healthcare practices, providing care recipients with opportunities for introspection, personal development, and a feeling of meaning.

THE LARGER CONVERSATION ON HEALING

Healing is not solely an individual journey; it occurs within the broader context of communities, cultures, and societal systems. Engaging in the larger conversation on healing, the author looks at other scholars' views on healing the whole person. She also looks at patients, caregivers, spiritual leaders, and healthcare professionals engagements in promoting shared understanding in the healing process and collective well-being. The author's intent is to discuss and acknowledge the interconnectedness of physical, emotional, and spiritual health while highlighting the importance of social support, cultural practices, and community resources. By situating individual care within this wider framework, healthcare providers can cultivate approaches that are both compassionate and contextually informed, ultimately promoting more sustainable and meaningful healing outcomes.

From the author's point of view, spiritual care plays an important role in helping the care recipient navigate through suffering. When a person is unwell, loses a loved one, or has a difficult healthcare experience, there is frequent emotional, psychological, and spiritual anguish. At such time, one is extremely susceptible, and medication alone should not be the only treatment; patients also require psychological and spiritual connection.[1] When one experiences some level of emptiness and confusion, the person's greatest need is the presence of someone who cares.[2] In a research study by Abu-El-Noor and Abu-El-Noor, healthcare providers are mandated by international authorities and organizations to attend to patients' spiritual needs, in addition to the national obligation.[3]

The spiritual caregiver places a higher priority on providing a loving presence and forming connections of support. By addressing one's spiritual and existential needs, offering emotional support, and helping the search for meaning and purpose in the face of suffering, spiritual care takes a compassionate and all-encompassing approach. Thus, in the field of healthcare, the importance of comprehending and treating the full person, including the body and spirit, has come to be better understood. So, "holistic care" has become a widely accepted idea, and according to studies, a holistic approach to care improves patient happiness and efficiency.[4]

Life crisis or suffering sometimes plunges one into the reality of one's human frailty.[5] The integration of spiritual care in healthcare acknowledges that individuals possess multidimensional aspects, including physical, emotional, social, and spiritual dimensions. Focusing on one's feelings, paying attention to what attracts one's attention, beginning to see the unique person that God loves, and recognizing the person's inner experience are what caring for

---

1. Abu-El-Noor and Abu-El-Noor, "Mapping the Road," 188.

2. Butler, *Caring Ministry*, 20.

3. Abu-El-Noor and Abu-El-Noor, "Mapping the Road," 191.

4. Roberts, *Professional Spiritual and Pastoral Care*, 23.

5. Butler, *Caring Ministry*, 20.

one's spiritual needs entails.[6] Recognizing and addressing these spiritual needs, which might also include religious convictions, moral principles, existential worries, and the search for meaning and purpose in the face of sickness is essential. Spiritual care has been discovered as a means to improve physicians' quality of life and the patient-clinician experience[7]. While other studies show that even among patients who are not religious, there is a considerable need for pastoral care on a spiritual level.[8]

Numerous studies have explored the impact of spiritual care on patient outcomes and overall healing. Findings consistently indicate that integrating spiritual care into medical treatments positively influences patients' physical and mental health. Thus, Swinton posits, "Religious spirituality has been positively associated with the alleviation of depression, anxiety, PTSD (post-traumatic stress disorder), schizophrenia, anorexia, and personality disorder."[9] People who receive spiritual care report reduced levels of anxiety, improved coping mechanisms, and increased overall satisfaction with one's healthcare experience.

Abdolkarimi, in "The Relationship Between Spiritual Health and Happiness in Medical Students During the COVID-19 Outbreak," reviewed other scholarly materials and found that spiritual health is so important that without it, other biological, psychological, and social dimensions of health cannot function properly, and the highest level of quality of life cannot be achieved.[10] This means that some sense of positive spirituality is a common human need, and everyone needs a sense of meaning and purpose, however one discovers or defines it. Thus, Swinton argues that spirituality is about whole-person care and a holistic way of viewing the individual.[11]

In our pursuit of healing the whole person, we turn our attention to the following themes and subthemes:

6. Butler, *Caring Ministry*, 20.

7. Finn and Roche, *Supportive Care Strategies*, 225.

8. Henderson et al., "Patient Religiosity and Desire," 81.

9. Swinton, *Finding Jesus in the Storm*, 33.

10. Abdolkarimi et al., "Relationship," 2.

11. Swinton, *Finding Jesus in the Storm*, 32.

Holistic Healing and the Role of Spiritual Care

Holistic healing is rooted in the understanding that health extends beyond the physical body, encompassing emotional, mental, social, and spiritual dimensions. Spiritual care, in particular, provides a vital pathway for addressing the deeper aspects of a person's well-being, helping individuals explore meaning, purpose, and connection in the face of illness or life challenges. This approach recognizes that each person's beliefs, values, and inner experiences profoundly influence their health journey. Integrating spiritual care into healthcare not only enriches the therapeutic relationship but also encourages self-reflection, inner growth, and a sense of wholeness, ultimately creating a more compassionate and comprehensive model of healing that honors the entirety of the human experience.

An approach to treatment known as holistic healing takes the full person into account, addressing not only physical ailments but also an individual's emotional, mental, and spiritual needs. It is a treatment philosophy that sets dissimilar and high expectations for quality of care, both for healthcare facilities and for all the interdisciplinary team.[12] This approach seeks to advance general harmony and well-being while acknowledging the interconnection of these dimensions. It entails determining and meeting the "spiritual needs" of patients, such as a patient's quest for inner tranquility, the meaning of life, the purpose of suffering, hope, a relationship with God, or "greater strength."[13]

Spiritual care, which recognizes the relevance of spirituality in the healing process, is an essential part of holistic healing. Regardless of a person's religious identity, spiritual care offers support, compassion, and understanding in one's spiritual journey. Thus, newer studies validate that the spiritual needs for chaplain care are indeed strong across patient populations, even in nonreligious patients.[14] It involves treating others as one would like to

12. Roberts, *Professional Spiritual and Pastoral Care*, 23.

13. Klimasinski, "Spiritual Care," 2.

14. Henderson et al., "Patient Religiosity," 81.

be treated if in the same situation. That is, showing sincere care, compassion, and acceptance, and helping others to rediscover meaning out of hopeless situations. It promotes a greater feeling of purpose and meaning in the life of the care recipient by encouraging one to explore ideas, values, and inner resources. "It is also of importance that an atmosphere of trust is created, without which the patient may not be able to reveal his/her inner experiences, fears and hopes."[15] Thus, patients who receive holistic care experience improvements in their mental and emotional well-being, which can lead to better management of physical symptoms and more positive treatment outcomes.

Significance of Spiritual Care

Spiritual care is an essential component of the whole person's care. Its significance stems from its ability to assist individuals as they navigate difficulties, disease, or life transitions, assisting them in discovering meaning, purpose, and inner peace. By addressing spiritual needs, healthcare providers promote resilience, hope, and a stronger sense of connection, which benefits both emotional well-being and general health. Integrating spiritual care into one's treatment plans enhances not only emotional and mental well-being but also overall health outcomes, reinforcing the understanding that complete healing involves attending to every aspect of the human experience.

The development of tailored religious support activities for accompaniment and emotional support that also aim to reaffirm spiritual beliefs and values, without necessarily involving forms and objects of worship, is significant in spiritual care. They are given by religious leaders as well as qualified health professionals and attempt to, among other things, encourage, reassure, and boost confidence, hope, and faith.[16] Sharing a profound closeness and connection, whether with God or one another, calls for brave

15. Klimasinski, "Spiritual Care," 6.
16. Dutra and Rocha, "Religious Support," 102.

vulnerability to reveal the core of one's being to another, as well as faith in the strength of relationships. It also needs a foundation of appropriate relationships and trust.[17] This significance lies in its recognition of the intrinsic spiritual dimension of human beings and its profound impact on overall well-being.

By attending to individuals' spiritual needs, beliefs, and values, spiritual care offers a holistic approach to healing, promoting emotional resilience, inner peace, and a sense of purpose and meaning in life. "It is an approach that should be shown to all service users and can be practiced by any member of the clinical team as a part of holistic care."[18] It plays a crucial role in healthcare settings by complementing physical and psychological treatments, facilitating coping mechanisms during times of crisis, and offering comfort and support in the face of suffering or end-of-life experiences. From analysis by Clyne et al., one of the most salient factors that arose was that, as participants felt validated and valued by healthcare professionals, which in turn supported one's desire to find meaning in one's remaining days and months, relationships with healthcare specialists, as part of good holistic patient-centered care, were meaningful to them.[19]

Spiritual care is inexpensive and does not call for specific equipment because it starts with a patient-centered, all-encompassing approach. The caring minister must not arrive armed with answers but with faith and the courage simply to be mindfully present to someone in pain.[20] Clyne et al. identified two main categories of spiritual care resources, which are the individual's personal resources and resources related to the professional support provided within the healthcare organization.[21] Simply discussing spirituality might offer spiritual assistance. This is far different from forcing someone to adopt one's religion or imposing one's

---

17. Baldwin, *Trauma-Sensitive Theology*, 74.

18. Kelly and Swinton, *Chaplaincy and the Soul*, 58.

19. Clyne et al., "Patients' Spirituality," e559.

20. Butler, *Caring Ministry*, 20.

21. Clyne et al., "Patients' Spirituality," e559.

views. While having a religious outlook does not make complaints go away, it does influence one's feeling of hope or despair.[22]

Incorporating Spirituality in Healthcare Settings

Incorporating spirituality in healthcare settings involves recognizing and valuing the spiritual dimension of patients' lives and integrating it into one's care. This includes understanding patients' beliefs, values, and religious backgrounds and offering respectful and non-judgmental support to address the care recipient's spiritual needs. Conversations should encourage patients to spend time thinking about what is important at this time and what type of interventions and situations should be avoided.[23] Healthcare professionals can engage in active listening and empathetic communication to foster trust and facilitate discussions about spirituality and its impact on health and healing. A better approach is the "support response," where the care provider urges the distressed person to talk more about whatever is bothering him/her. Often, allowing someone to process one's emotions is the most kind and uplifting support that the care recipient deserves.[24]

Additionally, creating a welcoming environment that accommodates diverse spiritual practices and providing access to chaplains, spiritual counselors, or support groups can further enhance the integration of spirituality in healthcare. Roberts asserts that to aid one in one's quest for healing, one must establish safe spaces where one can share one's experiences while being watched over by a caregiver who approaches this sacred moment with creativity, compassion, collaboration, and competence.[25] By doing so, healthcare providers can promote holistic well-being, emotional resilience, and improved patient outcomes while nurturing a sense of comfort, purpose, and connectedness for individuals facing

---

22. Klimasinski, "Spiritual Care," 11.

23. Finn and Roche, *Supportive Care Strategies*, 195.

24. Martelli, *Memory Eternal*, 133.

25. Roberts, *Professional Spiritual and Pastoral Care*, 122.

health challenges.[26] While being sensitive to the care recipient's cultural and religious preferences, Roberts argues that caregivers are the guides for those travelers who seem to have lost the way to a better health journey.[27]

Interdisciplinary Approach to Holistic Healing

A truly holistic approach to healing recognizes that no single discipline can address the full spectrum of a person's needs. Interdisciplinary care brings together healthcare providers from multiple fields: medicine, nursing, mental health, social work, spiritual care, and complementary therapies to collaborate in designing and delivering comprehensive care plans. By sharing knowledge, perspectives, and skills, these teams can address physical, emotional, social, and spiritual dimensions simultaneously, ensuring that treatment is personalized and well-rounded. This collaborative model fosters communication, reduces fragmented care, and empowers patients to participate actively in their healing journey, ultimately promoting more effective, compassionate, and sustainable outcomes. "Through interdisciplinary collaboration, the preferences, hopes, and values of the patient and caregiver can be integrated into the treatment plan, which is key in providing the delivery of optimal care."[28]

To address the physiological and psychological components of a patient's illness, medical experts collaborate with psychologists and counselors in the patient's plan of care because "there is a close body-mind relationship that must be explained, and the body and mind must be understood separately and in relation to each other."[29] Thus, diet plans created by nutritionists' support recovery by nourishing the body. Caregivers look at spiritual and emotional support, prayer, and yoga as examples of mindfulness techniques

26. Roberts, *Professional Spiritual and Pastoral Care*, 122.

27. Roberts, *Professional Spiritual and Pastoral Care*, 122.

28. Caecilie et al., "Interdisciplinary Collaboration," 1.

29. Joranger, *Interdisciplinary Approach*, 33.

that assist people in reducing stress, improving mental health, and developing a closer relationship with one's inner self. Consequently, an interdisciplinary approach to holistic care acknowledges that health is a dynamic interaction of several elements, with self as the autonomous center of self-reflection.[30] Therefore, when the team draws on the knowledge of numerous disciplines, one can experience dramatic alterations in one's overall well-being.

Myrhoj et al. studied the experiences and opinions of patients, caregivers, doctors, and nurses in relation to interdisciplinary collaboration during serious and complicated illness.[31] Despite its goal and success, the writers found that interdisciplinary relationships can sometimes be fragmented and uncoordinated due to challenges such as imbalance of authority, limited understanding of others' roles and responsibilities, or even gaps in communication. These can directly affect the contributions and roles of each profession during conversations and plans of care. Acknowledging that human health is complicated and interdependent, and that no one academic field can offer an all-inclusive solution, practitioners are encouraged to work together to develop an individualized treatment plan that tackles the underlying causes of health issues by using ideas from fields including medicine, psychology, nutrition, mindfulness, and alternative therapies.

Cultural Competence and Sensitivity

Cultural competence and sensitivity are vital to holistic healing, as they ensure that care honors the full complexity of individuals and the communities they come from. Every person's understanding of health, illness, suffering, and spiritual well-being is shaped by cultural background, traditions, and lived experience. When healthcare providers approach patients with openness, curiosity, and humility, they create space for those cultural perspectives to be expressed and respected. This commitment to understanding

30. Joranger, *Interdisciplinary Approach*, 40.

31. Caecilie et al., "Interdisciplinary Collaboration," 2.

diversity enhances communication, reduces barriers to care, and fosters deeper trust between patients and caregivers.

This subtheme is important because most people studiously avoid those who follow different moral standards, particularly in this day and age that celebrates diversity. Brooks asserts that some people tend to avoid individuals who hold different ideals than persons from different racial backgrounds.[32] One of the main challenges the Prophet Muhammed faced was convincing people to look beyond certain identity markers to see the heart and soul within an individual.[33]

By using examples from Western, Asian, and African contexts to demonstrate how culture affects counseling practices, pastoral counseling in multi-cultural contexts explores ways in which pastoral counseling reflects cultural preferences and suggests the need for respect for the universal, cultural, and unique aspects of all people.[34] Showing people sincere care, compassion, and acceptance and helping one to rediscover meaning out of despair is essential.[35] This is because spiritual caregiving is a professional practice of compassionate ministry that is most frequently done in secular institutions, seeking accommodation for all without the establishment of a specific religion.[36]

People today are seen as embodying several identities. These identities are all divinely intended and are given to humankind by God as a gift so that one can connect with creation's variety and richness.[37] The revelation of the kingdom of God as a new counterculture is the aim of the gospel. This new culture is characterized by a love for one another and a commitment to the virtues of patience, kindness, goodness, faithfulness, gentleness, and self-control.[38] As Muhammad Ali et al. posit, "I see beauty in all

---

32. Brooks, *Love Your Enemies*, 103.

33. Ali et al., *Mantle of Mercy*, 64.

34. Magezi, "Positioning Care," 3.

35. Kelly and Swinton, *Chaplaincy and the Soul*, 46.

36. Ali et al., *Mantle of Mercy*, 42.

37. Ali et al., *Mantle of Mercy*, 65.

38. Swinton, *Finding Jesus in the Storm*, 208.

our differences. As somebody who lived in places other than his native country for two decades, I grew accustomed to diversity in race, culture, language, and religion."[39] Therefore, Christians are called in Matt 22:37–40 to love God and to love one's neighbor as oneself, and John 13:34 says, "A new command I give you: Love one another. As I have loved you, so you must love one another."

While several healthcare institutions have recognized the importance of cultural competence and sensitivity in spiritual care, many hospitals have implemented the initiative to enhance the organization's care practices, taking into consideration the following.

Culturally Tailored Education

Culturally tailored education recognizes that individuals learn, interpret health information, and make decisions through the lens of their cultural values, language, and lived experiences. By adapting educational materials and communication styles to reflect these differences, healthcare providers can ensure that information is not only understood but also meaningful and relevant. When education is aligned with a person's cultural worldview, it enhances trust, promotes informed decision-making, and empowers individuals to take an active role in their healing. Ultimately, culturally tailored education strengthens the connection between patient and provider, supporting healing that is respectful, accessible, and truly person-centered.

If you would agree with me, the United States has become more diverse. It is now a place where all cultures are expected to be accepted and appreciated. This diversity is directly seen in governmental facilities, jails, hospitals, and clinics.[40] By understanding cultural nuances, providers can offer spiritual care that aligns with patients' beliefs and values, acknowledging personal biases, learning about different cultures, and being open to challenging one's assumptions to provide the best possible spiritual care.

---

39. Ali et al., *Mantle of Mercy*, 48.

40. Roberts, *Professional Spiritual and Pastoral Care*, 407.

Despite the developing clinical skills, medical trainees often do not receive sufficient formal instruction in humanism, professionalism, communication, and teamwork, areas that are essential but still underrepresented in many medical education programs.[41] Indeed, newer studies validate that the need for spiritual care is strong across patient populations, even in nonreligious patients.[42] While this is acknowledged as key to patient care, many nurses and other medical personnel do not feel adequately equipped to offer spiritual care due to insufficient skills and confidence.

So, Roberts points to the need for healthcare professionals to advance toward patient's overall well-being by actively working to understand the cultural origins and worldviews of the care recipient for the purpose of one's overall well-being.[43] By that, spiritual care professionals can develop a trustworthy and sympathetic relationship with patients that will promote a deeper connection by acknowledging and respecting peoples' cultural differences.

Respect for Religious Diversity

Respect for religious diversity is essential in holistic healing, as it affirms the dignity and individuality of each person's spiritual journey. Patients bring a wide range of beliefs, practices, and sacred traditions into the healthcare setting, and honoring these differences fosters trust, comfort, and a deeper sense of safety. When providers approach religious diversity with openness and genuine curiosity, they create space for patients to express what is meaningful to them, whether that involves prayer, ritual, sacred texts, community involvement, or quiet reflection. This respectful posture not only supports spiritual well-being but also strengthens the therapeutic relationship, reduces misunderstandings, and promotes care that aligns with a patient's values and worldview.

41. Finn and Roche, *Supportive Care Strategies*, 226.
42. Henderson et al., "Patient Religiosity and Desire," 81.
43. Roberts, *Professional Spiritual and Pastoral Care*, 408.

Spiritual practices of patients can be effectively included in care programs by spiritual caregivers who are competent. This may involve arranging for specific religious rituals, prayer spaces, or access to religious texts and resources. By including these components, healthcare ministers can build a more welcoming and encouraging environment, fostering a sense of comfort and belonging for patients during one's healthcare journey. In the provision of care, a caregiver will not ask why the person does not believe in God but will seek a way to establish a therapeutic relationship with the care recipient (patient, family, or staff).[44]

Sometimes, religious support is commonly characterized as religious or spiritual care and relates to rituals that seek the reconnection of the care recipient with God or with his beliefs and values.[45] Higher levels of religious belief are associated with greater levels of happiness and health.[46] The study of various religions, Islamic theological instruction with Muslim scholars, and the encouragement of introspective self-knowledge and growth necessary for compassionate care were three major facets of education at Hartford Seminary that helped Ali et al. develop an understanding of what it means to be a shepherd for everyone, regardless of the client's religious affiliation.[47] Thus, there is need for care providers to have knowledge of various religious traditions and be receptive to learning about new ideas and customs because caregivers who work in secular organizations provide care to religious and nonreligious persons. This is the reason why, at some hospitals, "pastoral care" is sometimes replaced with "spiritual care" to accommodate the needs of all.

Interpreter Services

Interpreter services is used to ensure that language differences never become barriers in the process of healing the whole person.

44. Klimasinski, "Spiritual Care," 9.
45. Dutra and Rocha, "Religious Support," 101.
46. Abdolkarimi et al., "Relationship," 2.
47. Ali et al., *Mantle of Mercy*, 38.

Effective communication is foundational to assessing needs, discussing treatment options, and exploring the spiritual and emotional dimensions of a patient's experience. Professional interpreters help bridge linguistic and cultural gaps, allowing patients to express their concerns, beliefs, and preferences accurately and confidently. By providing access to qualified interpreters, rather than relying on family members or ad-hoc solutions, healthcare settings promote dignity, reduce misunderstandings, and support informed decision-making. Ultimately, interpreter services uphold equity in care and strengthen the therapeutic relationship, enabling patients to fully participate in their own healing journey.

Interpreter services uses virtual technology to communicate and assess patient's overall need.[48] Many healthcare institutions now offer language interpretation services to assist patients who speak languages other than the dominant one. It is feasible, acceptable, and effective in a variety of clinical settings.[49] In Swedish Hospital, as in the entire nation, some patients come to hospital with limited English, and it is challenging for the nursing, medical, and other staff to provide the necessary treatment to them.[50] Additionally immigrants often arrive with illnesses not listed in any nursing, medical, or social work textbooks.[51] For instance, different from other countries, malaria is a common illness in Nigeria and the medications can be bought over the counter at any medicine store in Nigeria, but it is handled as a contagious and very serious disease in the United States and other countries. Given that malaria is a prevalent chronic health issue in Nigeria and that most people are aware of the disease's antecedent cause as mosquitoes, everyone is susceptible to contracting it and with less anxiety.[52] Understanding this and being able to communicate it effectively is essential in meeting the patient's need.

48. Sprik et al., "Chaplains and Telechaplaincy," 41.

49. Sprik et al., "Chaplains and Telechaplaincy," 41.

50. Roberts, *Professional Spiritual and Pastoral Care*, 408.

51. Roberts, *Professional Spiritual and Pastoral Care*, 408.

52. Ovadje and Nriagu, "Multi-Dimensional Knowledge," 10.

In a diverse community, patients generally come from different cultural and linguistic origins in a varied society, and excellent patient-provider communication is essential for precise diagnosis and treatment. Language barriers create challenges for clinicians in terms of obtaining an accurate patient history, care provision, discharge planning, and may also impact morbidity, mortality, and length of stay.[53] Beyond merely translating languages, interpreter services can also aid in navigating cultural quirks and preferences that could influence medical choices.

According to a systematic review conducted in the USA, professional interpreters were used, and patients who were cared for using professional interpreters had better health processes, outcomes, and utilization of health service.[54] A New South Wales-based study on communication in healthcare found that friends and family were prioritized above translators significantly in the emergency department.[55] Interpreter services guarantee that patients can appropriately explain their symptoms, worries, and medical history, and the medical professionals can effectively communicate information concerning diagnosis, treatment plans, and prescription instructions. A qualified interpreter acts as a cultural liaison, ensuring medical professionals are aware of any potential cultural obstacles that can influence diagnosis and treatment.

Community Engagement

Community engagement is vital in holistic healing. It recognizes that a person's well-being is shaped not only by clinical care but also by the strength and vitality of the community around them. When a person collaborates with individuals around them, like faith communities, cultural groups, and social networks, they gain a richer understanding of how other individuals cope with their difficulties and probably realize that they are not alone in life's struggles.

53. Duronjic et al., "Impact of Language Barriers," 1.
54. Duronjic et al., "Impact of Language Barriers," 2.
55. Duronjic et al., "Impact of Language Barriers," 2.

Life itself is all about connections to and of free, boundless, limitless, fluid energy that creates and maintains life. Divine energy holds human relationships to God, to each other, and to self together.[56] Within the larger context of cultural competency and sensitivity, community participation is an essential subtheme. It places a focus on how individuals and organizations may actively contribute to learning and respecting the many cultural backgrounds and requirements of local communities and people. Believers have a responsibility to spread God's beauty throughout their community. The dynamic aspect of human existence deals with how people perceive, communicate, and/or seek meaning, purpose, and transcendence, as well as how persons relate to the present, to self, others, nature, the significant, and/or the sacred.[57] Community engagement encourages discussion and cooperation.

A strong sense of community involvement in caring for one another is a key component of African spirituality. People are dependent on one another and on God. According to Prophet Muhammad, those who are compassionate toward God's creation are those God loves the most.[58] Ultimately, everyone has a deep need to be in touch with others. Even a self-centered person naturally wishes to have the kind of fiber that is willing to shoulder a fair portion of the agony and work because of this desire.[59] Thus, it is important for one to be able to provide spiritual care to those who may need it in various communities.

Engaging in a community challenges caregivers to develop competencies that enables individuals to function effectively within their immediate context and in a global setting.[60] It also gives them a circle of trusted friends who can pray together and share in many other meaningful activities.[61] A group is a tool to recognize and address one's own emotional barriers and limitations.

---

56. Baldwin, *Trauma-Sensitive Theology*, 126.

57. Connolly and Timmins, "Experiences Related to Patients," 2143.

58. Gilliat-Ray et al., *Understanding Muslim Chaplaincy*, 30.

59. Houselander, *Guilt*, 120.

60. Magezi, "Positioning Care," 3.

61. Gustafson, *Departure Dialogues*, 26.

Successful group members not only increase one's ability to relate to others but also gain more inner peace and have a much better grasp of one's own potential.[62] Thus, Martin Luther King Jr. posits, "All labor that uplifts humanity has dignity and importance and should be undertaken with painstaking excellence."[63] Accordingly, to feel dignified, one must be looked-for by others.[64] Therefore, community involvement promotes cross-cultural tolerance, fosters reciprocal learning, and eventually fosters a more peaceful and cohesive community/healthcare environment that values diversity and thrives on understanding.

Effective Spiritual Care

Effective spiritual care recognizes the unique inner world of each individual and responds with presence, empathy, and thoughtful attention to their beliefs, values, and sources of meaning. For spiritual care to be truly effective, it begins with listening, allowing patients to express their hopes, fears, questions, and spiritual concerns without judgment. This kind of care may involve supporting prayer, facilitating access to chaplaincy services, honoring cultural or religious rituals, or simply offering a compassionate, undistracted presence during moments of uncertainty. Through effective spiritual care, healthcare providers help patients build resilience, deepen their sense of connection, and find meaning in the midst of illness or transition.

Everyone has the capacity to recover and find happiness by transforming from a very deep place within oneself. Facilitating this inner change that in the end will transform the person's whole being and experience of life is what all effective care is about.[65] When patients are navigating the healthcare system, effective spiritual care is a patient-centered approach that tends to the person's

62. Martelli, *Memory Eternal*, 166.

63. Brooks, *Love Your Enemies*, 69.

64. Brooks, *Love Your Enemies*, 72.

65. George et al., *Holistic Healthcare*, 9.

emotional and spiritual needs. This process includes inquiring about spiritual concerns, offering sympathy, and fostering purpose and hope during illness and pain.[66] Recognizing and meeting the needs of the human spirit, including spirituality through compassionate relationships, should be the focus of spiritual care.[67] It is naturally related to greater patient well-being, happiness, hope, and appreciation.[68] It comprises encouraging patients and medical practitioners to have open and sincere discussions about their beliefs, morals, and existential concerns.

Spiritual care is effective when it recognizes the significant role that spirituality plays in a person's overall welfare while respecting the diversity of religious and spiritual traditions. Thus, an exploratory qualitative study engaged the question, "How do we develop a curriculum that facilitates reflection on psychological, moral, and spiritual experiences in caring for the critically ill and trains future professional caregivers in practices of self-care undergirding professionalism?"[69] Indeed, there is need to train healthcare professionals who actively listen, offer emotional support, collaborate with chaplains, and provide holistic treatment that respects a patient's spiritual preferences. Better spiritual well-being has also been linked to other areas of life quality, like psychological well-being and weariness. It incorporates the spiritual aspect into the patient's care strategy, guaranteeing that one's religious beliefs and practices are respected and considered alongside medical interventions.

Effective spiritual care acknowledges the value of patient autonomy, ethical issues, and cultural competence. Having spiritual or religious beliefs can help people to cope and find meaning and gain peace of mind in serious illness or when approaching death. It is a personal, subjective experience that is often motivated by the desire to comprehend the meaning of life and death.[70] The ul-

---

66. Yang et al., "Effect of Spiritual Care Training," 435.

67. Kang et al., "Meaning-Centered Spiritual Care," 3.

68. Kang et al., "Meaning-Centered Spiritual Care," 2.

69. Mitchell et al., "Developing a Medical School Curriculum," 728.

70. O'Brien et al., "Meeting Patients' Spiritual Needs," 183.

timate goal of spiritual care effectiveness is to improve the quality of healthcare overall, increasing patient satisfaction and promoting recovery and well-being. Thus, patients who feel or experience unmet spiritual needs report being less satisfied with the overall care and quality of treatment received.[71] "Patients with unmet spiritual needs are at increased risk of poorer psychological outcomes, diminished quality of life, reduced sense of spiritual peace and increased risk of depression."[72]

A tremendous deal of love is needed when providing such care, working with people's emotions and sexuality, helping the sick and insane in unlocking the darkest secrets, and patiently spending endless hours helping neurotic people let go of mistaken notions.[73] However, there are challenges to providing effective spiritual care, such as the diversity of beliefs among patients, the need for healthcare professionals to receive adequate training in spiritual care, excellent communication skills, interdisciplinary collaboration, cultural sensitivity, time constraints in busy hospital environments, and legal and ethical concerns. Reducing these disparities will be facilitated by gaining a better knowledge of the obstacles these minority populations face when in severe illness or near death.[74]

Challenges to Effective Spiritual Care

Providing effective spiritual care can be complex, as it requires sensitivity to diverse beliefs, the ability to navigate emotionally charged conversations, and the confidence to engage with topics that may feel deeply personal. Time constraints, heavy workloads, and limited training often leave healthcare providers feeling unprepared to explore spiritual concerns in depth. Differences in cultural or religious backgrounds between patients and caregivers

---

71. O'Brien et al., "Meeting Patients' Spiritual Needs," 183.

72. O'Brien et al., "Meeting Patients' Spiritual Needs," 183.

73. George et al., *Holistic Healthcare*, 9.

74. Mayeda and Ward, "Methods for Overcoming Barriers," 697.

can also create uncertainty about how to approach spiritual topics respectfully. In some settings, institutional policies or lack of inter-disciplinary collaboration further restrict opportunities for meaningful spiritual support. These challenges emphasize the need for ongoing education, supportive policies, and a culture that values spiritual well-being as an integral aspect of holistic care.

These difficulties can hinder the provision of holistic health-care that addresses the spiritual and emotional needs of one's care recipient. A study examined the effects of teaching nursing students two spiritual competency areas: spiritual patient care and spiritual awareness perceptions in oneself in a spiritual education courses. It asserts that "spirituality and spiritual needs are associated with cultural background and religious beliefs, and are important when evaluating nurses' spirituality."[75] Alternative training approaches and tools have been shown to be helpful in enhancing attitudes toward spiritual care and increasing awareness. Thus, addressing these challenges requires healthcare institutions to invest in training, foster a culture of respect and diversity, and develop clear policies and procedures for providing spiritual care. Some of the key challenges include the following.

Diversity of Beliefs and Practices

In a society where spiritual and religious customs are intricately knit together, the medical staff may encounter a range of belief systems, rituals, and values. This variety can make it challenging to provide treatment that is truly sensitive and appropriate to each person's unique spiritual demands. In a study, a nurse who describes herself as Christian expressed a feeling of ease caring for Christian patients and worried about upsetting someone who practiced another religion.[76] True, patients come from various religious and spiritual backgrounds, and one's beliefs and practices can be vastly different. Given that spirituality and spiritual needs are linked to one's

75. Yi-Chien et al., "Spiritual Education," 2.
76. Keall et al., "How Do Australian Palliative," 3202.

religious beliefs and cultural background, cultural context is crucial when assessing the spirituality of the care theme.[77]

Spiritual care integrates cognitive, affective, and behavioral dimensions, such as spiritual self-awareness, managing self-beliefs, respecting other's spirituality, providing spiritual care for patients, respecting cultural diversity, and guaranteeing the quality of spiritual care.[78] As such, care providers need to be well-informed and culturally competent to navigate the potentially dangerous terrain of other beliefs and behaviors without unintentionally offending or misunderstanding. Since better spiritual well-being was found to be related to such other aspects of quality of life as psychological well-being and fatigue, understanding that humans are spiritual beings, irrespective of one's religious background may be one of the strongest predictors for medical staff in providing spiritual care for patients.[79]

Lack of Formal Training

Many healthcare professionals lack formal training in providing spiritual care. Researchers have investigated why medical professionals, such as doctors and nurses, do not provide spiritual care more often, and one explanation for this could be insufficient training rather than self-reported obstacles such as a lack of time or private place.[80] Training medical staff by hospitals on spiritual care issues could have positive effects on patients' well-being, and inadequate training is the strongest predictor of rare spiritual care provision.[81] Therefore, creating training for medical professionals to offer religious assistance would be a proactive measure to guarantee that spiritual care is provided to the degree that patients and healthcare providers want and as required by federal regulations.[82]

77. Yi-Chien et al., "Spiritual Education," 2.
78. Yi-Chien et al., "Spiritual Education," 2.
79. Kang et al., "Meaning-Centered Spiritual Care," 2.
80. Yang et al., "Effect of Spiritual Care Training," 435.
81. Mitchell et al., "Developing a Medical School Curriculum," 728.
82. Mitchell et al., "Developing a Medical School Curriculum," 728.

In the past, healthcare and caregiving environments have prioritized the physiological aspects of care, leaving practitioners frequently unprepared to handle the complex and profoundly personal aspects of spirituality. Van de Geer et al., found that a practical and concise training program on spiritual care and pastoral care for healthcare professionals in teaching hospitals can improve staff attitudes and competencies, draw more attention to the spiritual dimension, and temporarily lower barriers to spiritual care for the medical staff.[83] A study by Yi-Chien et al. indicated that taking a spiritual education course was an effective means of improving nursing students' spiritual competencies for spiritual care and spiritual consciousness.[84] It demonstrated how multidisciplinary learning, interests, and spiritual competencies can be enhanced by a well-designed educational course.

When there is gap in spiritual care knowledge and skills, it can be a significant barrier to providing effective and sensitive support to individuals facing spiritual or religious challenges. To increase team members' ability to provide patients with the spiritual care that is required, training is badly needed.[85] To find out how new educational initiatives for healthcare personnel in spiritual care will impact patient care, there is a need to develop a model, put it into action, and evaluate its effectiveness. It is believed that because of the sensitive nature of spiritual care, extra training will be required for its implementation.[86] Thus, investing in formal education and training programs that teach medical personnel and other caregivers the skills and knowledge necessary to navigate a patient's spiritual world is crucial to bridging this gap.

83. van de Geer et al., "Multidisciplinary Training," 224.

84. Yi-Chien et al., "Spiritual Education," 5.

85. Kang et al., "Meaning-Centered Spiritual Care," 2.

86. van de Geer et al., "Training Hospital Staff," 744.

Communication Skills

Effective spiritual care requires strong communication skills to facilitate open, empathetic, and nonjudgmental conversations about patients' beliefs and values. It helps one to share what is in one's mind and heart without fear of criticism, contempt or defensiveness, as it could be detrimental to effective communication.[87] Healthcare professionals have been tasked with reassessing and introducing the complex concepts of spirituality and spiritual care, not just in hospice care but also in hospitals, other facilities, and home care.[88] These essential skills were not possible for some healthcare workers to possess, and some medical team members, like many others, take communication for granted. A study showed that discussing existential or spiritual issues with patients can lead to touchy subjects; however, good team communication and continuity of care needs to be balanced against the need for efficient collaboration and continuity of care.[89]

Since communication skills are essential for comprehending, honoring, and addressing an individual's spiritual and religious views, they can be a major obstacle to delivering good spiritual care. In a research study, several nurses stated that providing spiritual care requires effective communication skills.[90] When discussing questions of faith and spirituality, poor communication skills may cause misconceptions, insensitivity, or even accidental offense. "One hospital-based nurse reflected on how poor communication can make a difficult situation worse."[91] There is also a possibility for one to believe that an interpretation given to an event, behavior, or message is correct, even when it is in error.[92] To overcome this barrier, it is essential for healthcare personnel to receive training and ongoing education in communication techniques specifically tailored to fostering more effective and empathetic spiritual care.

87. Moitinho and Moitinho, *Dream Home*, 73.

88. van de Geer et al., "Training Hospital Staff," 744.

89. Keall et al., "How Do Australian Palliative," 3202.

90. Keall et al., "How Do Australian Palliative," 3202.

91. Keall et al., "How Do Australian Palliative," 3200.

92. Hills, "Overcoming," 99.

Legal and Ethical Concerns

Legal and ethical concerns play a crucial role in shaping how spiritual care is offered within healthcare settings. Providers must balance their desire to support a patient's spiritual well-being with the obligation to respect autonomy, confidentiality, and informed consent. This includes ensuring that spiritual conversations are patient-led rather than provider-led, avoiding any form of pressure and maintaining clear professional boundaries. Ethical practice also requires honoring religious diversity, protecting privacy, and recognizing when to refer patients to trained spiritual care professionals, such as chaplains. Additionally, healthcare institutions must comply with laws that safeguard patients' rights to their own beliefs and practices while preventing discrimination.

Balancing these ethical dimensions of care can be challenging. There may be legal and ethical considerations surrounding spiritual care, such as respecting a patient's right to refuse certain treatments or interventions based on one's spiritual beliefs. Any procedure involving people should be guided by the three moral principles of beneficence, fairness, and respect for individuals.[93] Thus, decisions about spiritual care may be complicated by issues with patient autonomy, informed consent, and the separation of church and state. In ethical procedures, written information is considered important, whether it is provided on paper or a mobile device.[94] In accordance with the informed consent principle, caregivers must provide participants with all the details required in decision processes[95] and ensure that the individual's rights and welfare are protected.[96] Finding the correct balance between upholding legal and ethical requirements and honoring an individual's spiritual beliefs can occasionally impede the comprehensive and tailored spiritual care that patients may require. This emphasizes

93. Tsosie et al., "Considering 'Respect for Sovereignty,'" 28.
94. Spatz et al., "New Era." 1.
95. Redman and Caplan, "Should the Regulation," 38.
96. Abay et al., "Rapid Ethical Assessment," 12.

the importance of having clear policies, training, and guidelines for navigating these.

Interdisciplinary Collaboration

Different healthcare professionals, including doctors, nurses, social workers, and chaplains, may have distinct specialties and approaches to dealing with spiritual issues. This uneven knowledge and application of spiritual care practices may lead to inconsistencies and gaps in the patient's support. Training in spiritual care can help with this self-awareness process.[97] Although most healthcare workers are not trained in the basic principles and techniques of spiritual care, the national practice guidelines highlight spiritual care as an area of care that can be provided by all healthcare providers in any context in which palliative patients are treated.[98] The target is the practical ability to provide spiritual, emotional and spiritual care to patient, family and staff.

Coordinating spiritual care with other aspects of healthcare, such as medical treatment and psychological care, can be challenging. Many medical professionals report a desire to provide spiritual support when a patient faces terminal illness, but, in reality, this happens less frequently than desired.[99] A more positive perspective on nursing care, spiritual care, and professional commitment is exhibited by higher spiritually healthy nurses.[100] Similarly, physicians are more likely to feel confident in engaging on spiritual matters with patients when one is comfortable in one's spirituality.[101] However, the competencies of medical staff as it relates to spiritual care are limited, despite its relevance in the healthcare sector; interdisciplinary teamwork can occasionally get in the way of providing effective spiritual care. Therefore, to overcome this challenge, there is need for healthcare facilities to

97. Mitchell et al., "Developing a Medical School Curriculum," 728.

98. van de Geer et al., "Training Hospital Staff," 744.

99. Mitchell et al., "Developing a Medical School Curriculum," 728.

100. Yi-Chien et al., "A Spiritual Education," 1.

101. Mitchell et al., "Developing a Medical School Curriculum," 728.

prioritize the integration of spiritual care into the larger interdisciplinary care paradigm.

Grief and End-of-Life Care

Grief and end-of-life care are integral components of holistic healthcare, requiring sensitivity, compassion, and a deep understanding of the emotional, spiritual, and cultural dimensions of dying. Effective care at this stage involves supporting patients and their families as they navigate loss, uncertainty, and the profound emotional challenges that accompany terminal illness or the death of a loved one. Spiritual care, counseling, and culturally informed practices can provide comfort, foster meaning-making, and help individuals reconcile with life transitions.

Patients with terminal illnesses may experience a range of physical, psychological, or spiritual symptoms and issues that can be upsetting and negatively impact one's quality of life. Providing spiritual care at such times can be emotionally and spiritually challenging for patients and healthcare providers. Patients with life-threatening diseases may develop a variety of symptoms and problems, which can be distressing and detrimental to one's quality of life.[102] Experts in providing round-the-clock care to terminally ill patients, such as hospice palliative care teams (HPCTs), are increasingly called upon to initiate spirituality-related conversations with patients and family.[103] Studies have shown that spiritual care often presents a challenge for HPCTs. As a result, healthcare providers are unable to provide patients with the spiritual care required for one's overall well-being.[104] Thus, to satisfy one of the most significant needs of human existence and provide spiritual care that is meaning-centered and oriented to one's spirituality, healthcare practitioners need to undergo some educational training for spiritual care skill acquisition.

102. Brinkman-Stoppelenburg et al., "Involvement of Supportive Care," 2899.

103. Kang et al., "Meaning-Centered Spiritual Care," 2.

104. Kang et al., "Meaning-Centered Spiritual Care," 2.

Given that a patient's anxieties, beliefs, and specific spiritual needs may change as the person approaches death, healthcare providers must constantly adapt to spiritual care approaches to meet one's spiritual needs. Studies show that most people would prefer to die as painlessly as possible, in the comfort of one's home, and surrounded by family and friends.[105] Thus, having a strong spiritual life may help one avoid feeling hopeless in the final stages of life, and receiving spiritual care is essential to receiving high-quality palliative care.[106] Accordingly, the significance of a patient-centered approach to spiritual care attuned to the changing needs of the care recipient during end-of-life experiences is underscored by the fact that failure to provide sensitive and adaptable spiritual support in these crucial moments can result in unmet needs and increased emotional distress.

Strategies for Overcoming Spiritual Care Challenges

Overcoming spiritual care challenges requires intentional strategies that promote understanding, collaboration, and adaptability. Education and training programs can equip healthcare providers with the knowledge and skills to address spiritual needs sensitively, while interdisciplinary collaboration ensures that expertise from chaplains, social workers, and mental health professionals is integrated into care plans. Open communication, active listening, and culturally responsive practices help build trust and respect with patients and families.

Overcoming barriers to effective spiritual care can also involve a combination of empathetic listening and understanding, cultural and religious sensitivity, spiritual care education, self-care, and a commitment to providing holistic support. The quality of the patient's support network plays a significant influence in predicting how well the patient will respond to therapy, highlighting the caregiver's critical position as a member of the patient's multidisciplinary

---

105. Mayeda and Ward, "Methods for Overcoming Barriers," 697.

106. Kang et al., "Meaning-Centered Spiritual Care, 2.

care team.[107] Firstly, healthcare providers should prioritize active listening and open communication with patients, regardless of one's faith or beliefs. Every medical practitioner will develop their own team communication strategy and demonstrate an active listening skill.[108] By creating a safe and nonjudgmental space, one is more likely to share one's spiritual concerns and needs.

The integration of spiritual care into nursing programs, seminars, and in-service training in the workplace as well as formal education for medical professionals were among the solutions suggested by participants in a study for overcoming barriers to providing spiritual care to heart patients.[109] Providing such care may contribute to one's overall health and well-being: quality of life, anxiety, and dejection may all improve. In addition, one's hospital stays and admission rates may decrease, and the overall treatment expenses may be reduced.[110] To help with the process of reconstructing and redefining social roles and family ties, caregivers require continuous support and education. Long-term caretakers are also less likely to be offered or seek medical support, such as mental health assistance, despite reporting a lower quality of life.[111]

Self-care is an important strategy for improving quality of care. The inclusion of self-care is among the core principles of training in palliative care medicine. Self-care has several facets, including elements related to the body, mind, soul, relationships, and environment.[112] A great deal of time and energy is expended on caring for a patient with an advanced illness. This coupled with lack of sleep and fears of the uncertain may bring heavy fatigue and exhaustion to the caregiver and may be compounded by the perception of overall distress.[113] The impact of burnout or, say, "compassion fatigue" can be spontaneous and goes well beyond

---

107. Finn and Roche, *Supportive Care Strategies*, 157.

108. Hills, "Overcoming," 100.

109. Abu-El-Noor and Abu-El-Noor, "Mapping the Road." 194.

110. Abu-El-Noor and Abu-El-Noor, "Mapping the Road." 197.

111. Finn and Roche, *Supportive Care Strategies*, 160.

112. Finn and Roche, *Supportive Care Strategies*, 223.

113. Finn and Roche, *Supportive Care Strategies*, 160.

the negative effects on healthcare professionals. It includes job discontent and intent to quit the profession. It lowers the quality of one's interpersonal relationships, impacts one's immune function, causes depression, decreased lifespan, and even suicide.[114] By fostering this collaborative approach, healthcare institutions can break down the barriers to effective spiritual care, ensuring patients receive holistic support that respects one's spiritual and emotional well-being, alongside physical health.

BIBLICAL PERSPECTIVES ON WHOLENESS

The practice of healing the whole person is deeply rooted in theological principles that recognize the interconnectedness of the physical, emotional, mental, and spiritual aspects of human existence. Drawing inspiration from diverse spiritual traditions, the theological foundation of this work asserts that human beings are not merely physical entities but created in the image and likeness of God and possess an inner dimension that craves purpose, connection, and divine existence. The Bible states, "God created mankind in his own image, in the image of God he created them; male and female he created them" (Gen 1:27).[115] This fundamental biblical teaching emphasizes that humans created in the image and likeness of God have intrinsic worth, dignity, and holiness, regardless of upbringing or circumstances. Bearing the image of God, it is required of humankind to do justice, to love kindness, and to walk humbly with God (Mic 6:8), laying down one's life for the other (1 John 3:16).

This understanding of humankind, created in the image of God (*imago Dei*), highlights the importance of treating every person with compassion, love, admiration, and healing as Jesus instructed: "A new command I give you: Love one another. As I have loved you, so you must love one another" (John 13:34).[116] It

114. Rehder et al., "Science of Health Care," 1097.

115. Wolde, "Separation and Creation," 639.

116. Casciaro, *St. John*, 147.

is this love for God and neighbor that motivates a person to be a compassionate caregiver and an ambassador of Christ. Accordingly, George et al asserted that to love is an inborn emotion, and a person cannot be taught to love other people if the person does not already love people.[117] Thus, the author opines that to become a therapist, one ought to love and care for and about people. Being a bad therapist will not serve the world.[118] Christ himself could have saved the world with a single tear or breath but chose to save it by taking on all of humankind's misery, uniting himself with the anguish of humankind, and making the ultimate sacrifice of his death on the cross.[119] In love, Christ laid down his life for his friends (John 15:13) and invited humankind to do the same.[120] The subheadings below further explore the theological framework for this study.

Compassionate Healing

Compassionate healing lies at the heart of holistic healthcare, emphasizing empathy, presence, and genuine care in every interaction with patients. It recognizes that healing extends beyond treating physical symptoms to addressing emotional, mental, and spiritual needs. By approaching care with compassion, healthcare providers foster trust, reduce suffering, and create a safe environment where patients feel seen, heard, and valued. Compassionate practices, such as attentive listening, validating emotions, and offering support tailored to individual beliefs and experiences, enhance the therapeutic relationship and contribute to meaningful, transformative healing. Ultimately, compassionate healing nurtures not only the patient but also strengthens the moral and emotional state of the patient's loved ones, promoting wellness on multiple levels.

---

117. George et al., *Holistic Healthcare*, 9.

118. George et al., *Holistic Healthcare*, 9.

119. Houselander, *Guilt*, 28.

120. Casciaro, *St. John*, 159.

Compassion and healing are major elements in the life and teachings of Jesus Christ. Jesus' actions of physical and spiritual healing are described in the New Testament, illustrating compassion for the whole individual. In the Gospel of Mark, Jesus made his mission to provide forgiveness and healing to the sick and sinners clear (Mark 2:17).[121] This claim emphasizes Jesus' goal of holistically healing people by attending to the person's spiritual and physical needs. In the Gospel of Matthew, Jesus showed compassion to the crowd and granted healing to the sick ones, exemplifying compassion for physical and spiritual needs (Matt 14:14).[122]

Spiritual care and holistic healing are grounded in this compassionate approach. Caring for the sick and broken is an expression of Christlike love, focusing on the individual's whole being, recognizing one's inherent worth, and providing support for one's spiritual journey. The psalmist rightly expressed how much God cares for his people and looks out for them, even in one's nothingness (Ps 8:3–8). So, Swinton posits, "The presence of Jesus does not pass, even if it may sometimes feel that way. We are not called to be happy; we are called to be joyful. Joy is the settled assurance that God is always with us and for us in all circumstances."[123]

Matthew 9:35 illustrates how Jesus went through towns and villages, educating people in synagogues, proclaiming the good news of the kingdom, and healing every disease and sickness the people were suffering from.[124] Undoubtedly, numerous stories of Jesus treating spiritual and emotional needs in addition to bodily illnesses are found throughout the Gospels. For instance, consider how frequently Jesus pardoned transgressions before and after curing medical ailments (Mark 2:1–12; Luke 7:36–50).[125] He demonstrated empathy for people's emotional and spiritual struggles (Matt 9:36, 11:28–30). These references provide a glimpse into the extensive healing ministry of Jesus, showcasing his compassion,

121. Olivi, "Commentary on the Gospel," 30.

122. Summers, "Matthew 14:13–21," 299.

123. Swinton, *Finding Jesus in the Storm*, 82.

124. Uytanlet and Kwa, *Matthew*, 105.

125. Healy, *Gospel of Mark*, 57.

authority over sickness, and the holistic nature of the care Jesus provides, addressing physical, emotional, and spiritual needs. In the end, Jesus' healing mission is a powerful illustration of God's mercy and love.

When four companions brought a disabled man to Jesus in Mark 2:5, Jesus said, "Son, your sins are forgiven." Jesus' healing experiences frequently include not just physical recovery but also emotional and sin forgiveness. This connection between physical healing and forgiveness highlights how spiritual and bodily health are intertwined in the ministry of Jesus. Furthermore, Jesus' interactions with people, such as the blind beggar Bartimaeus (Mark 10:46–52) and the woman with the issue of blood (Mark 5:25–34), demonstrate his attention to each person's particular needs, addressing not only the people's physical ailments but also their emotional and spiritual states.[126]

The Role of Faith

Faith can play a profound role in the process of healing, offering individuals a framework for meaning, hope, and resilience during times of illness, stress, or life transition. It provides a sense of connection to something greater than oneself, fostering inner strength and emotional stability. In healthcare, recognizing the role of faith allows providers to support patients in ways that honor their beliefs, values, and spiritual practices. Incorporating faith into care, whether through prayer, rituals, meditation, or simply acknowledging a patient's convictions can enhance coping mechanisms, promote mental and emotional well-being, and strengthen the therapeutic relationship.

Faith, as a theological foundation for spiritual care, serves as a profound and transformative force in the realm of holistic healing. At its core, faith represents a deeply held belief in something greater than oneself, often extending beyond the tangible and observable. St. Paul's letter to the Hebrews provided an assurance that

126. Olivi, "Commentary on the Gospel," 33.

faith is a conviction of things not seen but hoped for (Heb 11:1). Faith, prayer, and the guidance of the Holy Spirit bring comfort and healing to those suffering.[127] The Scripture talks about how faith in physical and spiritual healing may improve a person's overall well-being simply by trusting, and without faith, it is impossible to believe, to trust, and to please God (Heb 11:6). The emphasis on faith as a theological foundation can improve one's overall well-being by highlighting the intimate relationship between prayer, faith, and healing. This interaction demonstrates Jesus' recognition of the interconnectedness between faith, physical healing, and emotional well-being.

Within the Christian tradition, faith is seen as both believing that God can heal and having faith in his all-embracing plan for a person's life. With faith, whatever one asks in prayer will be received (Matt 21:22), for with God, nothing is impossible (Matt 19:26, Luke 1:37). Therefore, in spiritual care, a Christian is encouraged to trust in the Lord with all of one's heart, and not to lean on one's understanding (Prov 3:5–6). Thus, in all of life's journey, God makes straight the paths of those whose faith is in him. As in the Gospel of Mark 10:52 (ESV), Jesus said to the blind man, "'Go; your faith has made you well.' Immediately he recovered his sight and followed him on the way." Thus, faith is based on hearing, and hearing through the word of Christ (Rom 10:17).[128] These passages collectively emphasize the role of faith in the spiritual care and holistic healing process, illustrating the interconnectedness of faith, spirituality, and well-being. While author emphasizes the importance of faith in a patient's healing journey, it acknowledges the need for one to be open to the will of God. As in Mark 1:33–34, Jesus healed most of the people in the crowd, but not all.

127. Richardson, *Becoming a Healthier Pastor*, 67.

128. Adams, *Major Prophets*, 183.

Prayer and Ritual

Prayer and ritual draw people into a cycle of contemplation, relaxation, and connection that promotes overall healing. Through practiced gestures, spoken words, or moments of silence, these traditions create a sacred pause in which the mind settles, the body relaxes, and the spirit opens to meaning beyond the immediate moment. Prayer encourages inner dialogue and faith in something higher, whereas ritual gives structure and symbols to help people process emotions, mark transitions, and develop resilience. Together, they provide a steadfast framework for cultivating hope, presence, and integration throughout all aspects of the person.

Prayer is the movement of God into one's situation.[129] Many religious traditions place a high value on prayer and ritual as essential means of connecting with the divine, expressing one's beliefs, and discovering one's purpose in life. Prayer is seen as a means of opening a channel of communication with the divine. In prayer, one expresses one's thoughts, feelings, and desires to God, seeks guidance, and finds solace in times of need. "It is not simply a pious activity of the righteous, but rather a reaching out to God (Acts 17:27), who hears our sighs, our groans, and our laments."[130] It is a way to cultivate a personal relationship with God, "Our Father" (Isa 64:8–9). The majority of the world's religious systems practice prayer. People who pray use it to communicate with the "other," such as God, other people, or nature. There may be a set prayer hour each day or prayers to be offered for occasions like birth, death, illness, or celebrations in various religious traditions. Other traditions emphasize the spontaneity and in-the-moment nature of prayer.[131]

Prayer and the healing work of the Holy Spirit are indispensable for Christians.[132] Prayer restores one's connection with God, "for in him we live and move and have our being" (Acts 17:28).

129. Zylla, *Roots of Sorrow*, 127.

130. Zylla, *Roots of Sorrow*, 126.

131. Roberts, *Professional Spiritual and Pastoral Care*, 106.

132. Swinton, *Finding Jesus in the Storm*, 79.

During the days of Jesus' life on earth, Christ prayed and pleaded for God's help with intense sobs and tears to be delivered from death, and the prayer was heard by God (Heb 5:7–8).[133] So, Gustafson opines that "God gives human beings the freedom to pray with cries, tears, and words while remaining close to God who hears and promises to remain always with mankind."[134] Often, Jesus would withdraw to a lonely place to pray (Luke 5:16),[135] emphasizing the importance of prayer in Matt 6:9–13, when Christ teaches the disciples the Lord's Prayer. Thus, Gustafson asserts that Jesus prays for all mankind in all situations.[136] Likewise, healthcare professionals are called to pray sometimes for patients and families going through difficult times.

Patients across the religious spectrum strongly desire the chaplain's prayer in a time of need. James 5:14–15 (KJV) speaks to the power of prayer within a healing context. It suggests that if someone is sick, they should ask the church leaders to come pray for them and anoint them with oil in the Lord's name. Prayer offered with genuine faith will bring help and healing, the Lord will lift them up, and any sins they've committed will be forgiven. Praying together is a way to give voice to gratitude, suffering, hope, and need with a compassionate witness.[137] "Most importantly, prayer should not be imposed but should be offered in such a way that the patient/resident or family will sense no judgment if they decline."[138] This means the pastoral caregiver must not presume that a care receiver needs prayer. It must be offered and accepted.[139]

On the other hand, rituals, rooted in religious traditions, act as transformative tools for healing. These structured practices foster a sense of belonging and connection to the sacred, facilitating personal and communal healing. The story of the woman

133. Pink, *Exposition of Hebrews*, 262.

134. Gustafson, *Departure Dialogues*, 14.

135. Grun, *Jesus, the Image of Humanity*, 67.

136. Gustafson, *Departure Dialogues*, 34.

137. Henderson et al., "Patient Religiosity," 88.

138. Roberts, *Professional Spiritual and Pastoral Care*, 110.

139. Roberts, *Professional Spiritual and Pastoral Care*, 110.

who touched the hem of Jesus' garment in Mark 5:25–34 illustrates the healing power of ritual combined with faith, as such an act symbolized trust in divine healing. The Holy Communion, often known as the Holy Eucharist, the breaking of bread (Luke 24:35; Acts 2:42, 46; 20:7; and 1 Cor 10:16), is a significant ritual of oneness in God and denotes spiritual healing and nourishment in Christian theology. The apostle Paul stresses the value of participating in the Lord's Supper in 1 Cor 11:23–26, where believers remember Christ's sacrifice and get spiritual nourishment. Also, in the Jewish tradition, rituals such as the Passover Seder in Exod 12 and the Day of Atonement in Lev 16 are described as symbolic actions that reminded the Israelites of past history and renewed covenant with God.

Reconciliation

Reconciliation is the courageous work of restoring harmony within oneself, with God, and others. It begins with honest reflection, acknowledging hurts, misunderstandings, and the places where trust has been strained or broken. This process invites humility and compassion, allowing individuals to see their own wounds alongside the humanity of others. Reconciliation does not erase the past; instead, it opens a pathway to healing by transforming pain into understanding and division into renewed connection. As people mend these inner and outer fractures, they regain a sense of wholeness, dignity, and relational peace that strengthens their overall well-being.

The ministry of reconciliation emphasizes how crucial it is to repair bodily and spiritual wounds. The New Testament passage that most clearly centers on the theme of reconciliation is 2 Cor 5:17–21. The apostle Paul makes it clear that through reconciliation, a believer can become a "new creation" in Christ (2 Cor 5:17). To restore the brokenness brought on by sin, holistic healing looks to the transformative power of Christ's love, the Christ who was sent into the world to bring about peace by dying (Rom 5:10).[140] Thus, 2 Cor 5:18 states, "All this is from God, who reconciled us to himself through Christ and gave us the ministry of reconciliation." Therefore, achieving resilience and recovering from wounds, both traumatic and non-traumatic, requires tuning into the presence of the divine, the community's resources for care and support, and the calming, centered presence inside one another.[141]

Reconciliation involves seeking forgiveness, both from the divine and from fellow human beings. Second Corinthians 5:18–19 highlights the concept of reconciliation, that it is God who reconciled mankind to himself through Christ and gave humankind the ministry of reconciliation. This emphasizes that reconciliation is a divine act facilitated through Christ and extends to humanity, offering a pathway to holistic healing by repairing relationships with God and with one another. Thus, Jer 17:14 proclaims, "Heal me, Lord, and I will be healed; save me and I will be saved, for you are the one I praise." Accordingly, by Christ's wounds, believers are healed (1 Pet 2:24). Therefore, the beginning of human happiness is to know God, and keeping in mind that God alone can bring about healing, forgiveness, kindness, and an indescribable serenity.[142] So, knowing God as one true God and Christ Jesus is eternal life for all Christians (John 17:3), particularly, individuals navigating the complexities of life, illness, and suffering.

THEORETICAL PERSPECTIVES ON WHOLENESS

Wholeness emphasizes how humans are integrated, interwoven, and profoundly influenced by the relationships and circumstances in which they exist. Rather than considering health as the absence of illness, one can look at health or wholeness as a condition in which a person's bodily, emotional, mental, social, and spiritual components are in balance. Scholars from various disciplines see

140. Collins, "Jewish Source of Romans," 40.

141. Baldwin, *Trauma-Sensitive Theology*, 59.

142. Martelli, *Memory Eternal*, 172.

well-being as when all aspects of a person's life are acknowledged and encouraged, allowing people to take strength from meaning, connection, and resilience. It reminds us that wholeness is a continuous process, fostered by compassionate care, self-awareness, healthy relationships, and the presence of hope, even in the face of suffering.

Whole-person theory provide practical guidelines for how healing might occur in actual therapeutic settings. It emphasizes the need of collaboration among healthcare providers, incorporating spiritual and emotional support into medical care, and creating environments in which patients feel noticed and safe. Thus, caregivers are reminded that healing is more than just taking care of the physical; it is also about restoring dignity, hope, and significance. When wholeness is considered, it supports a style of care that respects the complexities of human life and promotes rehabilitation that touches the body, mind, and soul.

The integration of spiritual care into the healing process for those who are enduring physical, emotional, or psychological distress is emphasized in the domain of holistic healing. According to Roberts, "holistic healing" has become a widely accepted idea, and a holistic approach to care improves patient happiness and efficiency.[143] It is not also uncommon in the search for meaning and connection for individuals to talk about periods of struggle as well as times of peace and strength,[144] because the promise of God to preserve the lives of his children brings comfort (Ps 119:50). Thus, this theory involves integrating concepts from various disciplines, such as theology, psychology, and healthcare, for holistic care. The subheadings below explore this topic further.

Spiritual Ecology

Spiritual ecology invites us to understand our lives as woven into the larger web of the natural world. It highlights the way our emotional, physical, and spiritual health responds to the rhythms of the

143. Roberts, *Professional Spiritual and Pastoral Care*, 23.
144. Lydon-Lam, "Models of Spirituality," 19.

earth, its seasons, landscapes, and living systems. When we pause to breathe with the trees, listen to water, or simply feel the ground beneath our feet, we tap into a deeper sense of belonging and balance. This perspective encourages a relationship with nature that is both reverent and reciprocal. As we care for the environment, we indirectly nurture our own sense of wholeness, finding healing in the very world we help sustain.

This theory encourages individuals to connect with their inner selves, others, and the broader natural world for spiritual nourishment. The conviction that in moments of suffering, one is not alone but in spiritual communion with God and with the people of God, who share in the compassionate ministry of Christ in the world, brings comfort.[145] This theory challenges caregivers to examine a person's spirituality in terms of transcendence, growth, relational characteristics, values/beliefs, and meaning. Transcendence is "looking at the reality of human vulnerability, suffering, and evil."[146] But suffering is not to separate one from God (Rom 8:39). Rather, it tests the limits of one's connections to God and other people.[147] Thus, John 16:33 encourages believers to take heart and be assured God has overcome the world, no matter the troubles.

As part of spirituality, one may connect with things of this world, like family, friends, or nature, and with things not of this world (the divine, the universe, God) for one's spiritual and emotional health.[148] In providing care, one does not preach "family" and tell people what should be done. Rather, one starts where the care recipient is and just "comes alongside." It is a process of mutual discovery guided by one's understanding of how emotional systems function.[149] According to the holistic healing theory, treating the spiritual aspect alongside the physical and psychological ones might result in a more thorough and successful method of

145. Zylla, *Roots of Sorrow*, 140.

146. Schuhmann and Damen, "Representing the Good," 407.

147. Zylla, *Roots of Sorrow*, 126.

148. Lydon-Lam, "Models of Spirituality," 20.

149. Richardson, *Becoming a Healthier Pastor*, 123.

healthcare that fosters not only symptom relief but also personal development and inner peace. This concept of spiritual care transforms into a religious undertaking that aims to fulfill the deepest aspirations of the human soul by providing consolation, direction, and solace through times of adversity, pain, and illness.[150]

Maintaining a sense of the sacred relates to meaning in life and personal striving. Just as God is silently present to Jesus during his agony on the cross, he is equally silently present to everyone who suffers.[151] Like Jesus, Martelli emphasizes the need for caregivers to always remember that people going through suffering need love, not logic. "They need someone to sit and weep with them, not to present a sermon."[152] Thus, from this divine accompaniment, hope emanates. So, Rom 12:12 encourages believers to be joyful in hope, patient when afflicted, and pray fervently. As "the language of hope is rooted in God and God's infinite love."[153]

Spiritual Assessment Tools

Spiritual assessment tools help individuals and caregivers explore the beliefs, values, and practices that shape a person's inner life. These tools, ranging from guided questions to open-ended conversations, create space to understand what brings meaning, strength, and comfort to individuals, especially during times of illness or transition. By clarifying a person's sources of hope, beliefs, important rituals, and areas of spiritual struggle, one is better supported. Assessments reveal how spirituality influences coping, decision-making, and overall well-being. Used thoughtfully, they support more compassionate and personalized care, ensuring that healing attends not only to physical needs but also to the deeper flows of the human spirit.

---

150. Martelli, *Memory Eternal*, 45.

151. Ryan, *God and the Mystery*, 230.

152. Martelli, *Memory Eternal*, 45.

153. Zylla, *Roots of Sorrow*, 143.

It offers a methodical approach to investigating an individual's ideas, values, and existential concerns, and facilitates a more meaningful relationship between patients and healthcare professionals. "The importance of the spiritual assessment is understanding how or if a patient's spirituality affects their health care or how health care should be delivered."[154] Thus, Fitchett referenced Pruyser's study in support of his recommendation that the pastor's unique theological perspective, rather than the psychological worldview, should guide the spiritual assessment process,[155] since inspired pastoral acts are based on revelation from God that the caregiver either receives directly or is channeled through holy books or individuals.[156] So, the assessment tools should incorporate questions that can be used to understand the impact of spirituality on individual care plans.[157]

Here are some thoughtful, practical open-ended questions that could be used for spiritual assessment:

- *Do you mind telling me about the beliefs or practices that support you when you're facing stress or uncertainty?*

- *What spiritual or religious traditions play a meaningful role in your everyday life?*

- *What experiences, people, or practices help you feel supported or hopeful during challenging times?*

- *Do you mind sharing anything you've been wrestling with spiritually? For instance, doubts, questions, or concerns that might be influencing how you're feeling right now?*

- *What support system do you have, like family, friends, faith, or community?*

- *What rituals or reflective practices, such as prayer, meditation, music, or reading, feel important for your healing?*

154. Jones et al., "Spiritual Assessment," 417.
155. Fitchett, *Assessing Spiritual Needs*, 15.
156. Fitchett, *Assessing Spiritual Needs*, 12.
157. Jones et al., "Spiritual Assessment," 417.

- *How do you understand meaning or purpose in your life, especially when navigating illness or major transitions?*

- *What values or spiritual perspectives guide the way you make decisions about your care?*

- *In what ways can your care team honor and support the spiritual dimension of your healing experience?*

Holistic Healthcare Model

A holistic healthcare model views the person as an integrated whole, recognizing that physical health is deeply connected to emotional, social, and spiritual well-being. Rather than treating symptoms in isolation, this model encourages caregivers to consider the full context of a person's life. That is, one's relationships, beliefs, environment, and personal history. It values collaboration between patient and provider, emphasizing listening, shared decision-making, and individualized care plans that honor the person's unique story. By putting together medical treatment with supportive practices that nurture the mind and spirit, the holistic approach fosters deeper healing and a more balanced path toward healing the whole person.

According to a fundamental concept of spirituality, the body is sacred and the three (body-mind-spirit) are one; and without each one, the other cannot function properly. This perspective has been linked to actions that heal the whole person. It highlights how fostering spiritual resilience, coping mechanisms, and a sense of purpose can positively impact an individual's ability to heal and experience overall well-being. Speyer and Yaphe argue that, prior to addressing specific issues, solution-building must begin with imagining what the soul wants. Often, the ego needs security, significance, and a feeling of belonging, while the soul longs for wisdom, boldness, and transcendence.[158] Thus, Matt 16:26 (KJV) asks, "For what is a man profited, if he shall gain the whole world,

---

158. Speyer and Yaphe, *Applications*, 21.

and lose his own soul? Or what shall a man give in exchange for his soul?"

Collaborative Care Approach

The collaborative care approach brings together a team of health-care professionals who work in partnership with the patient to create a unified, comprehensive plan for healing. This model emphasizes communication, shared goals, and mutual respect among clinicians, caregivers, and the individual receiving care. Each team member contributes their unique expertise: medical, psychological, social, or spiritual, ensuring that no aspect of the person's well-being is overlooked. By fostering open dialogue and coordinated decision-making, the collaborative approach reduces fragmentation, improves continuity of care, and empowers patients to be active participants in their own healing journey.

Healthcare professionals are guides at the crossroads of where the care recipient's life situation meets one's life needs, values, personal qualities, and soul's purpose.[159] Medical professionals ought to foster a welcoming and accepting environment where individuals can discover and express their spirituality. For no one has the complete picture of the human person, yet all theorists contribute to it. Therefore, caregivers have much to gain from understanding other perspectives. Accordingly, Klimasinski argues that medical personnel can respond to the above needs outside the religious context by providing patients with respect and solicitude.[160] This theory views holistic health as encompassing a variety of healing approaches rather than just conventional medical treatments.

Narrative Medicine

The use of personal stories to comprehend and enhance health and well-being is a key component of narrative medicine, which serves

159. Speyer and Yaphe, *Applications*, 17.

160. Klimasinski, "Spiritual Care," 2.

as a theoretical underpinning for holistic treatment and spiritual care. This theoretical method acknowledges that a person's story, which is made up of one's experiences, convictions, and values, greatly influences how one sees sickness and recovery. For instance, people have described families as the reason why things are the way they are.[161] "The labels we use to describe our family members can say as much about us as about them. Our labels for others reveal the position we have taken in life vis-à-vis those people."[162]

In the context of spiritual care, narrative medicine prompts healthcare providers to listen attentively to patients' stories, not only to diagnose medical conditions but to comprehend the spiritual dimensions that contribute to one's overall health and provide comfort. Thus, one can take a lesson from one's own human sorrow and gently share the good news of God's nearness with the care recipient, who is grieving and alone,[163] while referencing God's promise to never leave nor forsake one (Heb 13:5). By acknowledging and engaging with these narratives, practitioners can offer more patient-centered and empathetic care that addresses not just physical symptoms but the broader context of an individual's life.

The significance of storytelling as a therapeutic tool that aids a person in making sense of one's experiences and giving one's recovery process direction is recognized by the discipline of narrative medicine. Reflection on this hidden experience reveals three yearnings of the afflicted: the longing to be seen, the yearning for a community of belonging, and the need to be understood.[164] The relationship between medical professionals and patients is strengthened by this approach, which encourages candid conversation and collaborative exploration of personal narratives, moving toward a one-on-one relationship, and being able to open up to the caregiver and talk about disturbing issues.[165] When used in conjunction with spiritual care, narrative medicine facilitates a greater

---

161. Richardson, *Becoming a Healthier Pastor*, 37.

162. Richardson, *Becoming a Healthier Pastor*, 38.

163. Zylla, *Roots of Sorrow*, 118.

164. Zylla, *Roots of Sorrow*, 120.

165. Richardson, *Becoming a Healthier Pastor*, 49.

understanding of the existential and spiritual aspects of a patient's life by medical practitioners, enabling them to integrate these aspects into a holistic healing process. By incorporating narrative medicine into spiritual and religious care, healthcare providers can forge stronger connections with patients, tailor interventions to align with the person's unique narratives, and contribute to a more comprehensive and meaningful healing journey.

Biopsychosocial-Spiritual Model

The biopsychosocial-spiritual model is a comprehensive approach that combines biological, psychological, social, and spiritual elements. It offers a solid theoretical perspective on wholeness. In this theoretical approach, when an individual is faced with problems, the person tries to cope with some internal religious resources, which are likely to influence the person's health outcomes.[166] Using this model of patient care as a framework, caregivers examine the ways patients can be supported physically, psychologically, socially, and spiritually.[167] Engel et al. acknowledge the intricate relationships between biological, psychological, and social elements in understanding illness and its man-agency.[168] The biopsychosocial-spiritual model fosters a deeper knowledge of the individual within one's cultural and spiritual environment by emphasizing a patient-centered approach that addresses the entirety of human experience through the incorporation of spiritual care.

This holistic perspective acknowledges that health is more than just the absence of illness; rather, it is a dynamic balance across various domains. In spiritual care, the biopsychosocial-spiritual model recognizes the importance of purpose, meaning-making, and connection in the healing process. From a physical perspective, a holistic model of biopsychosocial-spiritual care should include an emphasis on a healthy lifestyle, including regular sleep,

166. Anim et al., "African Cultural Values," 179.
167. Vermette and Doolittle, "What Educators Can Learn," 2062.
168. Anim et al., "African Cultural Values," 179.

physical exercise, healthy eating, and a connection with a spiritual being.[169] For one cannot achieve anything when away from God, because God is the vine and humans are the branches. It is in God that one bears bountiful fruit (1 John 15:5). He, the Lord, lights up the path of those who love him (Ps 119:105). So, if one identifies with a faith tradition, it is good to consider attending services in a consistent manner and aligning work with intrinsic values, such as through advocacy, community engagement, or peer support.[170] Medical personnel can engage with patients in a more compassionate and culturally sensitive manner by addressing the spiritual side of one's health, and one can modify interventions to target the patient's overall welfare.

Following the biopsychosocial-spiritual theory, rather than focusing on the patient's diagnosis, the healthcare provider should consider the experience of the individual seeking care as a human being deserving of compassion. Of course, there has been a lot written on approaches to treating the "whole person" and acknowledging a patient is a person with goals, a family, relationships, and culture, not just about the diagnosis.[171] With such consideration, the caregiver and the care recipient can all receive God's grace, no matter how fused and problematic the situation may be.[172] Therefore, let one's thinking, feeling, and behavior be less determined by what others expect and more by what makes sense in life, to self, to others, and to God, based on one's beliefs and values.[173] Encouraging gratitude, fostering a growth mindset, and promoting appreciative inquiry are all well-supported by scholars as effective ways to enhance well-being and enhance career development.

---

169. Vermette and Doolittle, "What Educators Can Learn," 2062.

170. Vermette and Doolittle, "What Educators Can Learn," 2063.

171. Vermette and Doolittle, "What Educators Can Learn," 2062.

172. Richardson, *Becoming Healthier Pastor*, 66.

173. Richardson, *Becoming Healthier Pastor*, 66.

Existential Well-Being Model

The existential well-being model emphasizes the fundamental relationship between existential problems and general well-being, serving as a strong theoretical perspective for healing the whole person. This model suggests that addressing existential issues has a vital role in enhancing an individual's feeling of completeness, and it acknowledges the importance of people finding meaning and purpose in life. Many patients turn to organized religion for answers to questions about what it means to live and die; others turn to some spiritual views that are not connected to any one religion for guidance.[174] But the commonly held assumption is that individuals more involved in religion are more likely to be passive or avoidant in the approach to dealing with diseases and other life situations.[175]

Despite one's health state, using a coping technique more frequently—that is, having a positive attitude and not having an anxiety disorder—results in an independent association with a stronger feeling of meaning, tranquility, and purpose in life.[176] Therefore, the existential well-being model helps healthcare professionals better understand what a patient has been through and encourage them to consider issues of purpose, values, and meaning-seeking in the context of spiritual needs.

Education and Training

While providing care, one might regularly run into unexpected storms and situations for which one is unprepared. Effective holistic healthcare requires that practitioners not only master clinical skills but also cultivate an understanding of the spiritual, emotional, and social dimensions of patient care. Education and training programs should integrate interdisciplinary approaches, emphasizing empathy, active listening, cultural competence, and

174. Sulmasy, "Biopsychosocial-Spiritual Model," 1931.
175. Sulmasy, "Biopsychosocial-Spiritual Model, 1936.
176. Sulmasy, "Biopsychosocial-Spiritual Model, 1931.

reflective practice. This prepares healthcare providers to recognize and address the diverse needs of individuals, fostering healing that extends beyond the physical body. Ongoing professional development, mentorship, and experiential learning opportunities ensure that caregivers remain responsive to evolving patient needs and the broader principles of whole-person care. According to Richardson, caregivers need to learn how to steer the patient's boat through harsh seas and help the care recipient to develop the skills that self-differentiation offers.[177]

Comprehensive education in spiritual care ensures practitioners develop a nuanced understanding of diverse spiritual beliefs, cultural practices, and existential concerns. In addition to producing technically sound and clinically competent doctors, medical education aims to foster the development of physician healers who can offer patients the best possible comprehensive care.[178] When healthcare practitioners are educated and trained in the theoretical underpinnings of spiritual care, they become more skilled. Additionally, this makes it easier to incorporate concepts of holistic treatment into more expansive healthcare systems.

This theoretical perspective on wholeness embraces the interconnectedness of mind, body, and spirit as a holistic model of healthcare. It integrates the biopsychosocial-spiritual framework, draws inspiration from existential models of well-being, and values the efficacy of narrative medicine. For instance, in critically ill patients, lower levels of psychological distress, such as suicidal ideation, depression, and hopelessness, are associated with higher levels of spiritual well-being.[179] Most often, one's feeling is shaped and labeled within one's life experiences.[180] This comprehensive approach turns spiritual care into a customized, intricate practice that is an art and a science and significantly contributes to people's total healing.

---

177. Richardson, *Becoming a Healthier Pastor*, 148.
178. Vermette and Doolittle, "What Educators Can Learn," 2064.
179. Sulmasy, "Biopsychosocial-Spiritual Model," 1931.
180. Richardson, *Becoming a Healthier Pastor*, 64.

CONCLUSION

It is clear from the author's point of view that introducing spiritual care in medical settings can benefit patients in several ways, including lowering stress and anxiety levels and enhancing general well-being. The significance of understanding the holistic nature of recovery, which recognizes the interconnectedness and impossibility of separating the physical, emotional, and spiritual facets of a patient's existence were emphasized. Some religious traditions' texts and teachings place a strong emphasis on the connection of all things, compassion, inner harmony, and completeness. Thus, as healthcare continues to evolve, it is imperative that healthcare organizations recognize the profound impact of spirituality on patients' well-being and recovery.

As healthcare systems continue to serve diverse populations moving forward, a commitment to cultural competence and sensitivity in spiritual care becomes increasingly important in delivering holistic care that addresses the spiritual and emotional needs of patients. It is important that healthcare organizations across the world continue to fund staff training in cultural sensitivity and competency, embracing diversity, and respecting patients' spiritual beliefs through a more inclusive and compassionate atmosphere, where patients feel valued and respected throughout their healthcare experience. By incorporating spiritual care into healthcare protocols and fostering a holistic approach, healthcare facilities can aim at promoting healing on all levels of care.

3

———

Reintroducing the Method

WHEN TRANSITIONING FROM AN academic dissertation to *Healing the Whole Person*, it was necessary to reevaluate how the methodology would be presented. In the original study, this chapter was extensive, technical, and structured to fulfill stringent academic standards, including step-by-step procedures, participant selection criteria, interview protocols, and in-depth analytical frameworks. While necessary for scientific assessment, this level of information might be daunting for readers looking for practical insights into holistic treatment.

Therefore, rather than removing this chapter entirely, it was summarized and made concise to preserve its educational value while maintaining readability. This is because methodology is more than a procedural account; it provides the foundation for understanding how the findings were derived, why they are credible, and how they can be applied in real-world healthcare and pastoral settings. By summarizing the methods, readers can grasp the research design, ethical considerations, data collection, and analysis processes without being lost in technical details.

Thus, the methodology chapter serve purposes such as follows:

- Demonstrating the rationale behind the study design: readers learn how the holistic healing intervention was structured, highlighting principles that can guide similar programs in healthcare, nursing, or pastoral care.

- Showing the rigor of qualitative research: even in condensed form, the chapter communicates that the findings presented later are evidence-based, systematically gathered, and thoughtfully interpreted.

- Providing transferable knowledge: beyond procedural description, readers gain practical lessons about planning, implementing, and evaluating interventions that support emotional, spiritual, and physical well-being.

Essentially, this chapter serves as both a road map and a learning aid. Understanding the technique allows readers to better appreciate the results, interact critically with the findings, and evaluate how the lessons can inform the healing of the whole person. As you read this chapter, consider it not just a description of "what was done" but also a source of information and direction, demonstrating how careful planning, ethical rigor, and reflective practice work together to make holistic care effective and meaningful.

HOW THIS BOOK WAS DEVELOPED

Caring for cardiac patients frequently focuses on the physical body, while the emotional and spiritual elements of recovery remain in the background. The author sought to investigate those ignored components and to pose a simple but essential question: What happens when spiritual and emotional care coexist with medical treatment?

To address that, the author carefully listened to the experiences of healthcare workers at Swedish Hospital in Chicago. Through questionnaires, interviews, and observation, the collected voices and ideas helped form the holistic therapeutic approach offered in this book.

The author used guiding questions like

Research Question 1: How do you address the emotional and psychological aspects of healing alongside the physical aspect of healing?

Research Question 2: How can support networks, such as those in the family and community, be more effectively tapped into to promote spiritual and emotional healing for cardiac care patients?

This chapter also explored the intervention design and the implementation of the intervention design.

DESIGNING THE INTERVENTION

To investigate the spiritual and emotional landscape of patient care, author employed a qualitative technique, which prioritizes depth over quantity and seeks significance beneath the surface of people's statements. Qualitative research is ideal for spiritual and pastoral work because it invites tales, nuances, and experienced experiences that do not usually appear in charts or statistics. "In most qualitative research design, the degree to which interviews and observations are structured varies."[1] This approach enables a deep understanding of people's experiences, perceptions, and behaviors. It investigates the character of one's experience, including its quality, various manifestations, contexts in which these experiences emerge, and viewpoints from which it can be observed.[2]

The intervention itself was straightforward; the author gathered the experiences of cardiac-care staff through open-ended questionnaires, interviews, and direct observation and let their insights guide the development of a holistic healing model. Participants were chosen intentionally, not at random, because the goal was to speak with people who could provide important insight into the emotional and spiritual requirements of cardiac patients. The value came from their actual experience rather than their quantity.

1. Devers and Frankel, "Study Design in Qualitative Research," 268.
2. Busetto et al., "How to Use and Assess," 3.

How the Plan Unfolded

The overall process took about ten weeks. Here is the flow in plain language:

- *Recruitment* began with staff from the hospital's cardiac units. After initial conversations and emails, nine participants agreed to take part, a number well within the typical range for qualitative studies seeking depth and saturation.

- *Consent and explanation* came next. Every participant received clear information about what the study involved, their freedom to withdraw, and how their privacy would be protected.

- *Questionnaires* were sent ahead of interviews so participants had time to reflect.

- *Interviews* were scheduled at their convenience, usually in their offices or quiet conference rooms.

- *Data collection* included conversation, observation of non-verbal cues, and the researcher's notes. With permission, interviews were audio-recorded and transcribed.

- *Data analysis* involved reading, rereading, and coding the transcripts and written responses to identify repeating themes, patterns, and important nuances.

- *Findings and recommendations* emerged as the final step.

Though a formal table guided the weekly plan, the heart of the process was simply listening carefully and honoring what participants shared.

Research Process and Ethical Care

Since this investigation took place within a healthcare setting, careful ethical oversight mattered. Permission was granted by Swedish Hospital's Institutional Review Board and later by Liberty University's IRB. Participants were offered full knowledge about the purpose of the study, how information would be handled, and how their confidentiality would be protected.

All digital data were stored on password-protected, encrypted devices. Physical documents were later shredded, and identifying information was removed from transcripts. Collected data will be destroyed three years after the study's completion—enough time for publication and follow-up work, yet short enough to safeguard participant privacy.

Participants and Sampling

The broader population included about one hundred and fifty staff members across the cardiac care units of Swedish Hospital. From this group, nine participants, men and women ranging in age from twenty-five to seventy-five volunteered to participate. Purposive sampling was performed, which means volunteers were chosen based on their firsthand experience caring for cardiac patients. This technique ensured that the study represented actual, grounded experience rather than abstract theory.

Participants contributed through

- open-ended questionnaires,

- semi-structured interviews, and

- the researcher's observational notes.

Together, these sources painted a complex picture of how spiritual and emotional care currently fits, or fails to fit, into clinical practice.

Interview Protocols

The interviews unfolded over several weeks, generally two or three per week. Before each conversation, participants had already completed the questionnaire, giving them time to think and reflect. A semi-structured format was used, meaning there were guiding questions, but conversations were allowed to move naturally.

Participants could elaborate, pause, reflect, or share unexpected insights. This flexibility is what makes qualitative interviewing so powerful; it lets the hidden or unspoken parts of experience surface at their own pace.

The questions focused on the emotional, spiritual, and relational dimensions of patient care:

- how they support patients beyond medical treatment,

- how families and communities are involved,

- what challenges they notice, and

- where they see gaps that spiritual or emotional care could fill.

Interviews were recorded (with permission) and transcribed using Otter.ai. The transcripts were later shared with participants for accuracy.

Data Collection

The conventional approach, which is frequently employed by qualitative researchers, entails an in-person, one-on-one interview, during which a guided dialogue is recorded and the researcher makes note of any nonverbal cues.[3] Data were collected through questionnaire and interview, scheduled to last about thirty minutes (maximum). Otter.ai, a transcribing application, aided in transcribing all interviews. Updated transcripts were secured in a password-protected computer to preserve participants' confidentiality.[4] The participants provided information based on the five open-ended research questions and some probing questions during the face-to-face interview. By being open-ended, the questions were designed as nondirective explorations that allowed for participants' choice of words, context, descriptions, and meaning regarding one's experiences.[5]

3. Billups, *Qualitative Data Collection Tools*, 6.
4. Cabral et al., "Challenges to Implementing," 4.
5. Cabral et al., "Challenges to Implementing," 7.

This method permits a profound comprehension of individuals' experiences, perceptions, and behaviors with quality, different manifestations, the context in which they appear, or the perspectives from which they can be perceived.[6] This aspect of the semi-structured interview strategy is crucial to its effectiveness; the researcher must be flexible to discern what qualifies as a "lead" and which line of inquiry should follow as the discussion develops.[7] This method of data collection generally includes data in form of words rather than numbers.

Gathering and Working with the Data

Each interview lasted about thirty minutes. Observations about tone, hesitation, emotion, and non-verbal cues were recorded in notes, providing important context for interpreting the verbal responses.

The goal wasn't to count responses but to understand them, to notice what kept coming up, where there was tension or longing, and what might point toward a more integrated model of care.

The analysis involved

- reading every transcript closely,

- identifying themes and subthemes,

- noticing repeated patterns, and

- capturing unexpected insights.

This interpretive work required not only technique but attentiveness, intuition, and pastoral sensitivity, a different kind of analysis than statistical testing, but one no less rigorous.

6. Busetto et al., "How to Use," 3.
7. Billups, *Qualitative Data Collection Tools*, 9.

IMPLEMENTING THE MODEL

With the data gathered, the next step examined how a model of holistic healing could be developed and implemented within hospitals setting. The intervention centered on recognizing that health is more than the absence of disease; it is physical, emotional, and spiritual well-being woven together.

Implementing the intervention model required

- assessing the spiritual needs of the patient population,

- understanding staff capacity and challenges,

- identifying goals for holistic care, and

- shaping a process that honored the lived experience of both patients and caregivers.

Here, creativity played an important role. Of course, qualitative work frequently requires the researcher to listen intently, identify patterns, and convey meaning in ways that are true to both the data and the people behind it.

Setting the Interview

Every interview was held in a venue chosen by the participant: a private office, a quiet conference room, a serene nook of the hospital, or somewhere that felt comfortable. These settings fostered an environment in which participants could openly discuss their experiences with patients' emotional and spiritual needs.

A triangulated approach, combining surveys, interviews, and the researcher's notes, provided a more complete picture of each participant's perspective. Audio recordings and transcripts ensured accuracy, while the safe setting contributed to authenticity.

Participants

The participants in this study came from the cardiac-care team at Swedish Hospital in Chicago, a group whose daily work already reflects a blend of clinical skill, compassion, and patient advocacy. Their perspectives were especially valuable because they interact with patients at the physical, emotional, and spiritual levels of care. The group included

- nurses, who spend the most time at the bedside and are often the first to notice a patient's emotional or spiritual needs as they unfold in real time

- physicians, whose medical decision-making is increasingly influenced by an awareness of the whole person, not just the present condition;

- a case manager, who helps coordinate treatment plans and sees how emotional or spiritual concerns can shape a patient's progress, discharge planning, or support systems;

- a unit assistant, who supports patients and staff in day-to-day operations and often catches the human details that fall outside the formal chart;

- a chaplain, who brings spiritual presence, prayer, listening, and pastoral support, and who often accompanies patients and families through moments of fear, grief, or ethical uncertainty.

Ethical Considerations

The intervention design was conducted rigorously in compliance with the ethical standards governing research involving human participants. Before the study began, Swedish Hospital's stakeholders gave ethical approval. This approval process ensured the protocols, participant rights, and study design complied with recognized ethical standards. Thus, protecting participants from adverse consequences associated with one's involvement in a research project, namely physical or moral suffering.[8] In addition to participant's voluntary participation, all participants signed the

8. Gaudet and Robert, *Journey Through Qualitative Research*, 5.

informed consent document, which was sent to participants in soft and hard copy format. This document outlined the goals of the study, any potential risks and benefits, and the promise of anonymity. The possibility to withdraw from the study at any moment without consequence was made clear to participants. Accordingly, Gaudet and Robert assert, "You must also explain how you will respect the right to anonymity and informed consent during the key steps of the project: the recruitment, the data collection, the archiving of data and the presentation of results."[9]

Ethical considerations during the intervention focused on maintaining the privacy and confidentiality of participants. All data collected through interviews and questionnaires were anonymized and securely stored in a password-protected laptop to prevent unauthorized access. Additionally, the intervention prioritized the well-being of participants. Check-ins with the participants before and after the data collection were implemented to address any emerging ethical concerns promptly, considering the need to treat every participant fairly.[10] Member checking, also known as respondent validation, is the process of following up with study participants to inquire whether the findings align with one's perspectives.[11] Overall, the ethical framework established for this intervention aimed to uphold the dignity, autonomy, and well-being of all participants involved, fostering a research environment that prioritized ethical conduct and the responsible advancement of healthcare practices.

Analyzing the Findings

This served as the road map for making sense of the information gathered and ensuring that the research questions were answered with clarity and rigor. At its heart, data analysis is about bringing order and meaning to a large, sometimes unwieldy collection of

9. Gaudet and Robert, *Journey Through Qualitative Research*, 5.

10. Gaudet and Robert, *Journey Through Qualitative Research*, 5.

11. Busetto et al., "How to Use," 7.

qualitative material generated throughout the research process.[12] The plan guided how key elements were identified, how the data were cleaned and prepared, and which analytical strategies would be used. Just as importantly, it laid out how the findings would be interpreted in light of the study's objectives. A well-designed analysis plan doesn't just organize work, it strengthens the credibility and transparency of the entire project.

For this project, the qualitative analysis centered on data collected during a holistic healing intervention at Swedish Hospital in Chicago. Interviews with care team members were recorded and transcribed using Otter.ai to ensure an accurate and verbatim account of participants' responses. Before the deeper analysis began, the material was condensed and summarized, a necessary step that also comes with the inherent risk of losing some pieces of the original context. As Gaudet and Robert point out, trying to describe qualitative analysis purely in theoretical terms is difficult; the process is lived, iterative, and shaped by the researcher's engagement with the data.[13] Transparency about that process becomes one of the strongest indicators of validity.[14]

The analysis itself involved manually coding the transcripts to identify emerging themes, subthemes, and patterns. Open coding allowed early ideas to surface, insights into participants' experiences, challenges, and perceptions of the holistic healing approach. Focused coding then sharpened these insights, helping distinguish core themes from supporting ones and deepening our understanding of the intervention's impact. The combination of audio recordings and transcripts enriched this process, preserving not just the words but also the tone, emotion, and emphasis conveyed during the interviews. The transcripts were prepared verbatim, with attention to behavioral cues when relevant.[15] Throughout the analysis, returning to the original audio via Otter.ai provided a reliable way to confirm meaning and maintain contextual

---

12. Sensing, *Qualitative Research*, 194.

13. Gaudet and Robert, *Journey Through Qualitative Research*, 5.

14. Sensing, *Qualitative Research*, 224.

15. Busetto et al., "How to Use," 4.

accuracy. By blending these approaches, the study aimed to offer a full, authentic view of how the holistic healing intervention shaped the experiences of healthcare professionals, patients, and families at Swedish Hospital.

Summarizing the Intervention Implementation

The preliminary findings during this implementation phase of the holistic healing intervention offered compelling insights into the initial impact of integrating spiritual and emotional care into conventional medical practices. Across the care team, there appears to be a notable shift in awareness and attentiveness to the holistic needs of patients, with participants expressing an increased recognition of the interconnectedness between physical, emotional, and spiritual well-being. The interdisciplinary team meetings have emerged as crucial forums for collaborative discussions, fostering a more cohesive approach to patient care that goes beyond traditional medical parameters. Early indications suggest that the intervention has prompted enhanced communication among care team members, enabling them to address the multifaceted dimensions of patient health more effectively.

According to participants in this study, patients also exhibit positive responses to the integrated care model, with anecdotal reports suggesting a heightened sense of comfort and support. The initial stages of the intervention have revealed instances where patients felt more heard and understood, particularly in relation to one's emotional and spiritual concerns. This aligns with the overarching goal of the intervention, emphasizing the importance of patient-centered care that acknowledges and incorporates the diverse needs of individuals. While these preliminary findings are promising, the ongoing analysis in chapter 4 will delve deeper into the complexities of the intervention's impact, examining both positive outcomes and potential challenges that may emerge over the course of the study.

4

———

From Design to Discovery

HAVING OUTLINED HOW *HEALING the Whole Person* was developed, through carefully designed interventions, structured research processes, and thoughtful participant engagement, now let's turn to the heart of the study, the results. The previous chapter laid the foundation, describing the intervention design, data collection, and analytical approach, showing how each step was deliberately used to capture the lived experiences of patients, families, and the healthcare providers. This chapter builds on that foundation, presenting what the research revealed about the integration of spiritual and emotional care into conventional medical practices.

The findings highlight the profound ways in which holistic healing can transform both patient experiences and healthcare delivery. Through interactions, challenges, and successes, the multidimensional nature of healing was made clear. Spiritual and emotional care was not merely an added service; it became a lens through which participants viewed the entire healing process, emphasizing interconnectedness between the body, mind, and spirit.

The results are organized into five overarching themes, each highlighting critical elements of holistic care, as shown below:

1. *Holistic Care*—Exploring the recognition of patients as complete beings, where physical, emotional, and spiritual needs are addressed in tandem.

2. *Support System/Network*—Examining the role of family, friends, and community in reinforcing emotional and spiritual well-being.

3. *Effective Communication and Collaboration*—Demonstrating how interdisciplinary teamwork and open dialogue enhance patient-centered care.

4. *Barriers and Factors Affecting Integration*—Identifying challenges that limit the seamless incorporation of spiritual and emotional care into routine practice.

5. *Impact of Spiritual and Emotional Care Interventions*—Highlighting tangible outcomes on patient recovery, satisfaction, and overall well-being.

Each theme will be explored in depth, integrating participant voices, observational insights, and reflective analysis. Together, these findings offer a compelling narrative of what happens when healthcare embraces the whole person, reminding us that healing is not just a clinical process but a deeply human one. By linking the structured methodology from chapter 3 with the lived experiences documented here in chapter 4, the author provides readers, whether students, practitioners, or general audiences, with a road map for understanding the need to heal the whole person.

As you read this chapter, you will notice a persistent emphasis on the relational, emotional, and spiritual aspects of care. These findings do not exist in isolation; they are linked with institutional procedures, interdisciplinary teamwork, and the human journeys of both patients and caregivers. By the end of this chapter, the findings will not only illuminate the efficacy of holistic interventions but will also prompt us to reconsider what it truly means to heal the body, mind, soul, and spirit.

BACKGROUND OF THE STUDY
AND COLLECTIVE RESULT

A key component of patient-centered treatment is the incorporation of spiritual care into holistic healing techniques. This approach, which has its roots in the Swedish Hospital's dedication to meeting each person's unique requirements, acknowledges the significant influence spirituality may have on one's general well-being. In a bustling urban environment where patients may face various stressors, incorporating spiritual care becomes imperative for fostering resilience and promoting holistic healing. This initiative aligns with the hospital's philosophy of treating patients as full individuals with distinct spiritual and emotional aspects, rather than only as medical problems.

This concept extends beyond conventional medical treatments to encompass a comprehensive approach that nurtures the mind, body, and spirit. In other words, "spirituality is the connection between the different parts of the human being (body, mind and soul)."[1] Therefore, patients are provided with a supportive environment where one's personal values, religious beliefs, and existential concerns are recognized and integrated into one's recovery process through the provision of spiritual care. Through various means, such as meditation rooms, chaplaincy services, or cooperative dialogues with healthcare personnel, Swedish Hospital endeavors to establish environments that respect and nurture a sense of consolation and ease for the patients and the patient's relatives.

Research on the effectiveness of spiritual care in healthcare setting has shown promising results, indicating its positive impact on patient outcomes, satisfaction, and overall well-being. This mounting body of evidence underscores that commitment to holistic health, which is demonstrated by its commitment to integrating spiritual care into its operations. Swedish Hospital promotes a healing environment that supports patients' overall well-being in

---

1. Hvidt et al., "What Is Spiritual Care?," 7.

addition to improving the quality of patient care by acknowledging and treating the spiritual aspects of health.

The author is concerned about the need for healthcare organizations to focus not only on physical ailments but also on patient's spiritual, mental, and emotional needs for the purpose of holistic healing. Thus, the purpose of this investigation is to develop and implement a model of holistic healing for integrating spiritual and emotional care alongside physical treatment for cardiac care patients. The following research questions were used to initiate this study and gain knowledge in this area:

Research Question 1: How do you address the emotional and psychological aspects of healing alongside the physical aspect?

Research Question 2: How can support networks, such as those in the family and community, be more effectively tapped into to promote spiritual and emotional healing for cardiac care patients?

Research Question 3: How can healthcare institutions create an environment that fosters collaboration and communication among multidisciplinary teams, including physicians, nurses, chaplains, social workers, and mental health professionals, to provide holistic healing for patients?

Research Question 4: What are the existing barriers and factors that affect the integration of spiritual and emotional care into the cardiac care journey, both within healthcare institutions and among healthcare providers?

Research Question 5: How can integration of spiritual and emotional care interventions into the Annual HealthStream Education impact patients' holistic healing process?

Prior to beginning the data collection, the author obtained permission from Liberty University's IRB. Participants included members of the care team, who were within the age bracket of twenty-five to seventy-five, and up to five years' experience and above in the healthcare profession at Swedish Hospital. All participants were intentionally selected using purposive sampling to ensure that the criteria for selection were met. Thus, Gaudet and Robert assert, "In assembling your project, you will have established selection criteria for your population in order to identify the relevant people to observe, interview or gather documents from."[2] Of the one hundred and fifty staff, the researcher struggled to find nine participants who met the criteria and were willing to participate in the study. The nine participants responded to the questionnaire using Google Forms, and responses were submitted to the researcher using the same method.

During the recruitment process, the researcher discovered that some staff who met the criteria were not comfortable participating in spiritual care matters, and some others were constrained by time. Each participant was assigned a double alphabetic pseudonym name, ranging from A to T. Accordingly, Gaudet and Robert assert that care must be taken to use a system of symbols or pseudonyms to identify all participants in all the collected data to maintain anonymity.[3]

DATA ANALYSIS

Data analysis is the process of bringing order, structure, and meaning to the complicated mass of qualitative data that the researcher generates during the research process. This requires some creativity in placing the raw data into logical, meaningful categories to examine data in a holistic fashion.[4] It needs to be done methodically and with a research mindset, which means one should always challenge one's own logic.[5] During data collection, Otter.ai was used to transcribe the interview and Google Forms was used to collect participants' responses from the questionnaire. Transcribing each of the nine interviews using Otter.ai software gave the researcher the opportunity to preserve the participants' words,

---

2. Gaudet and Robert, *Journey Through Qualitative Research*, 8.

3. Gaudet and Robert, *Journey Through Qualitative Research*, 15.

4. Sensing, *Qualitative Research*, 294.

5. Gaudet and Robert, *Journey Through Qualitative Research*, 7.

which enhanced the data's richness. The participants were sent a copy of the transcript through email, so each participant could have the opportunity to make any necessary revisions, but none of the participants asked for a change. The transcripts revealed themes and categories, which the researcher further explored using manual coding to find themes, subthemes, and multiple responses.

The qualitative data were analyzed using the thematic analysis structure as a framework to interpret data based on five themes. A methodical and popular way to extract themes from qualitative data is thematic analysis.[6] The findings presented in charts focused on addressing the research questions of the study based on the data collected using open-ended questions. The data were coded and tallied to ascertain the response frequencies and percentages using the multiple-response model, where each coded response had the opportunity of reoccurring multiple times. Coding, according to Graham, means "recognizing that not only are there different examples of things in the text but that there are different types of things referred to."[7] The results were further presented point by point to address the research questions of the study.

Theme 1: Holistic Care

Holistic care is a comprehensive model of caring, which is believed to be the heart of the science of nursing. The philosophy behind holistic care is based on the idea of holism, which emphasizes that for human beings, the whole is greater than the sum of its parts and that mind and spirit affect the body.[8] This approach seeks to advance general harmony and well-being while acknowledging the interconnection of these dimensions. The respondents emphasized that care must be holistic to ensure a comprehensive emotional and spiritual healing process. According to the respondents, "Care must be holistic in nature. Thus, it is essential that pastoral

---

6. Smith et al., "A Qualitative Study Exploring Therapists," 578.

7. Gibbs, Analyzing Qualitative Data, 3.

8. Tjale and Bruce, "A Concept Analysis," 46.

care givers must work with other healthcare team members for the healing of the patient" (Respondent AB). In this study, holistic care includes the use of collaborations, communication, participatory approach, family, and friends.

Collaboration

In this context, collaboration refers to the process where individuals from different health professions work together to positively impact patient care. It involves integrating knowledge, methods, and perspectives from multiple academic disciplines to address complex problems or issues. According to Klimasinski, through interdisciplinary collaboration, the preferences, hopes, and values of the patient and caregiver can be integrated into the treatment plan, which is key in providing the delivery of optimal care.[9] The respondents viewed that collaboration among the healthcare providers will be of utmost importance for the holistic emotional and spiritual healing process.

Communication and Participatory Approach

Communication among multidisciplinary healthcare teams was emphasized. A respondent said,

> As a CCU Nurse, I listen to patient's complaints and address their needs as they arise. I try to understand and accept their behavior as they are experiencing discomforts and provide the appropriate treatment they need. I also offer emotional support through spending time talking to them, and giving words of comfort acknowledging their culture and beliefs, and make referral for follow ups where and when necessary. (Respondent EF)

Respondent QR amplified the need for communication in the patient's healing process:

9. Klimasinski, "Spiritual Care," 1.

We might then discuss briefly how emotional and psychological factors can negatively impact healing. I will also continue questioning in an effort to empower them to address some of their distress themselves, such as what sorts of activities help you when you feel less frustrated or anxious. What helps you to calm down when you feel anxious? When patients seem to be at a total loss I might ask, have you ever tried meditating or taking a walk or watching a religious program? Sometimes I will ask if they might want to try a meditation or deep breathing, or reading with them at that time to help them experience the potential benefits of taking action on their own.

Family and Friends

The role of family and friends in the emotional and spiritual healing process cannot be overemphasized. The respondents viewed the role of family, friends, and loved ones to be very crucial in ensuring holistic care. According to Respondent MN, "For me personally, I have relied on the support of my closest family members. Having people who care about me has helped me so much in the past to get through my most trying times. Just knowing I am not alone has always given me hope and cheered me up." Respondent KL assured, "Personally, through prayer and family/friends. I lean on family (parents mostly) and partner when needed. And then after advice is offered up, I tend to pray on it." These responses succinctly underscored the relevance of family and friends in ensuring holistic healthcare for cardiac patients.

Theme 2: Support System/Network

Support systems and networks in this context refer to various strategies for providing emotional and spiritual support, such as active listening, understanding patient behavior during discomfort, offering words of comfort, and acknowledging cultural beliefs, cultivating positivity, relying on prayer, family, and friends.

The researcher expected a strong support system would promote emotional and spiritual healing.

Emotional and Spiritual Healing

Emotional and spiritual healing is a psychological care. It encompasses various practices, including counseling, prayer, meditation, and rituals, tailored to an individual's spiritual beliefs and values.[10] To achieve emotional and spiritual healing, the support networks must be functional, as opined by the respondents. One of the respondents emphasized that "every human being needs a support system. This could impact the healing process. A patient healing could be faster when the person feels connected to loved ones" (Respondent AB).

> The presence of the family and community, like the church, help promote spiritual and emotional healing in a way that they are the support group that provide strength and gives hope and uplift the spirit, especially when patient needs to undergo a major procedure like open heart. (Respondent EF)

For Respondent IJ, "I think first, a person needs to have a good support system to be able to utilize them. If one is established, I myself find that this, most often than not, tends to happen on its own. A great support system almost always, in my opinion, is associated with a promotion of spiritual or emotional healing, regardless of the type of patient." The respondents strongly associated emotional and spiritual healing with effective support systems/networks in healthcare services.

Theme 3: Effective Communication and Collaboration

To foster collaboration and communication among multidisciplinary teams, including physicians, nurses, chaplains, social workers, and mental health professionals, to provide holistic

10. Kelly and Swinton, *Chaplaincy and the Soul*, 58.

healing for patients, communication has to be effective. Effective communication entails engagement, cooperation, and information sharing among multidisciplinary healthcare units and teams to ensure holistic healing of patients. The respondents perceived that effective communication and collaboration can be achieved among healthcare providers.

> The healthcare institutions can create an environment that foster collaboration and communication among multidisciplinary teams, including physicians, nurses, chaplains, social workers, and mental health professionals, to provide holistic healing for patients by delivering consistency of care through daily rounds, assessment of physical, mental, emotional, spiritual, and social needs of patients and addressing their needs, providing important information about their test results and treatment, calling family for update of care and patient's condition and most especially by acknowledging and respecting diversity of culture. (Respondent EF)

Respondent AB maintained that, "as noted above, healthcare professionals must work together to foster the total healing of the person. This process includes collaborations that is engaged with open communication."

Theme 4: Barriers/Factors Affecting Integration

Aware that the most well-designed interventions also face obstacles, this theme explores the challenges encountered in integrating spiritual and emotional care into conventional medical practice. This theme points out the existing barriers and institutional factors that affect the integration of spiritual and emotional care into the cardiac care journey, both within healthcare institutions and among healthcare providers. They include but are not limited to lack of awareness and education on spiritual and emotional care and inherent institutional factors.

Lack of Awareness and Education on Emotional and Spiritual Care

Owing to the fact that caregivers provide support to people with various mental and physical health conditions in residential and nursing care facilities throughout the world,[11] a respondent affirmed that awareness and education on emotional and spiritual care was a major barrier. The respondent argued that

> lack of education and training about spiritual care among nurses, lack of time due to short staffing, individual barriers like lack of interest in nursing, negative perception of religious beliefs, problems in nurses' family relationship, and financial problems can be a barrier. (Respondent EF)

More so, Respondent QR said there is "limited understanding of spiritual care in healthcare. Lack of education of the support chaplaincy can provide religious prejudice against faith in a healthcare setting."

Institutional Factors

The respondents were equally of the view that some inherent institutional factors affected the integration of spiritual and emotional care into the cardiac care journey, both within healthcare institutions and among healthcare providers. Factors such as lack of good support system, lack of clear institutional policies, high level of provider burnout, lack of time due to short staffing, lack of education and training about spiritual care among nurses, and lack of continuity affected the integration of spiritual and emotional care. Accordingly, Smith et al. argues that the experiences of individuals giving spiritual care interventions have received relatively little consideration.[12]

11. Smith et al., "Qualitative Study," 576.
12. Smith et al., "Qualitative Study," 576.

Theme 5: Impact of Spiritual and Emotional Care Interventions

The respondents emphasized that spiritual and emotional care interventions have helped in creating awareness and understanding of the need for spiritual care, creating an environment of hope and support, improving care interventions, overcoming decades of pharmaceutical driven practices, and promoting seamless chaplain services in healthcare institutions. According to Respondent MN,

> Integrating spiritual and emotional care interventions into a hospital's continuing education program either in person or online can help increase awareness and understanding of the spiritual and emotional factors that impact a person's overall health. It can help caregivers develop strategies for assessing these factors and then to learn strategies and techniques to assist themselves and their patients to address these aspects of healing. . . . Integrating spiritual and emotional care into HealthStream education benefits the patient and the healthcare worker. I think it is important to create an environment of hope and support. Recognizing physical needs within the healthcare setting is only one part of a patient's journey. (Respondent KL)

In conclusion, the holistic care strategy needed to treat the psychological and emotional components of recovery in addition to the physical ones in cardiac care units is highlighted by this thematic analysis. Key themes include holistic care, support systems/networks, effective communication, barriers and factors affecting integration, and impacts of spiritual and emotional care interventions.

Table 1: **Thematic Analysis of Patient's Spiritual,
Physical, Social, and Emotional Healing**

Themes	*Subthemes*	*Codes*
Holistic Care	Collaborations	Caregivers must work with other healthcare teams
		Pay attention to spiritual and physical needs
		Listen to patient's complaints
	Communication and Participatory Approach	Understand and accept their behavior
		Offer emotional support
		Cultivate positivity by having a positive mindset
		Think positively
		Pay attention to the patient
		Ask the patient questions
		Psychosocial support
	Family and Friends	Use of closest family members
Support Systems/ Network	Emotional and Spiritual Healing	Feels connected to loved ones
		Improves the outlook on the patients' conditions
		Impacts the healing process positively
		Cultural and societal understanding and spiritual care for the patient
		Promotes emotional and spiritual healing

Themes	Subthemes	Codes
Effective Communication	Collaboration and Communication	Work together as a team
		Open communication
		Acknowledge and respect diversity of culture
		Holistic healing for patients
		Team members collaborate
		Communicate with all care team
		Involve family, friends and patient in every decision
		Medical record charting
		Use of chaplaincy
Barriers and Factors Affecting Integration	Awareness/Education on Emotional and Spiritual Care	Lack of education and training about spiritual care among nurses
		Negative perception of religious beliefs
		Patients' varying comfort levels
		Lack of spirituality
		Language and culture barriers
		Lack of awareness/education on emotional and spiritual care
	Institutional Factors	Lack of good support system
		Lack of clear institutional policies
		High level of provider burnout
		Lack of time due to short staffing
		Lack of education and training about spiritual care among nurses
		Lack of continuity

Themes	Subthemes	Codes
Impact of Spiritual and Emotional Care Interventions		Creates awareness and understanding of the need for spiritual care
		Creates environment of hope and support
		Improves care interventions
		Overcomes decades of pharmaceutical driven practices
		Promotes seamless chaplain services

Research Question 1

How do you address the emotional and psychological aspects of healing alongside the physical aspect of healing?

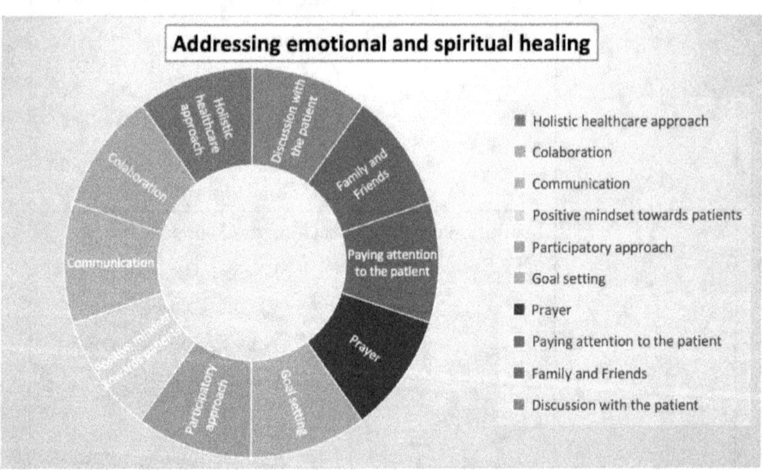

Figure 1. Addressing Emotional and Spiritual Healing

*Summary of Points for Addressing Emotional
and Psychological Aspects of Healing*

The findings presented in figure 1 showed the respondents perception of how to address the emotional and psychological aspects of
healing alongside the physical ones. Based on the findings, a large
proportion of the respondents (40 percent) perceived that emotional and psychological healing can be better addressed using a holistic
healthcare approach (see appendix A). One of the respondents said,
"Healthcare must be holistic in nature. Thus, it is essential that pastoral caregivers must work with other healthcare team members for
the healing of the patient" (Respondent AB). A holistic healthcare
approach seeks to advance general harmony and well-being while
acknowledging the interconnection of these dimensions.

More so, 30 percent of the respondents perceived that emotional and psychological aspects of healing can be better addressed
with the use of family and friends. One of the respondents com-
mented on this significance "personally, through prayer and fam-
ily/friends. I lean on family (parents mostly) and partner when
needed. And then after advice is offered up, I tend to pray on it."
Another respondent said, "For me personally, I have relied on the
support of my closest family members. Having people who are
care about me has helped me so much in the past get through my
most trying times. Just knowing I am not alone has always given
me hope and cheered me up" (Respondent KL).

Other approaches suggested by the respondents in addressing emotional and psychological healing were the participatory
approach, asking questions to the patient, collaboration, communication, positive mindset toward patients, prayers, goal setting,
and discussion with the patient.

Research Question 2

How can support networks, such as those in the family and community, be more effectively tapped into to promote spiritual and
emotional healing for cardiac care patients?

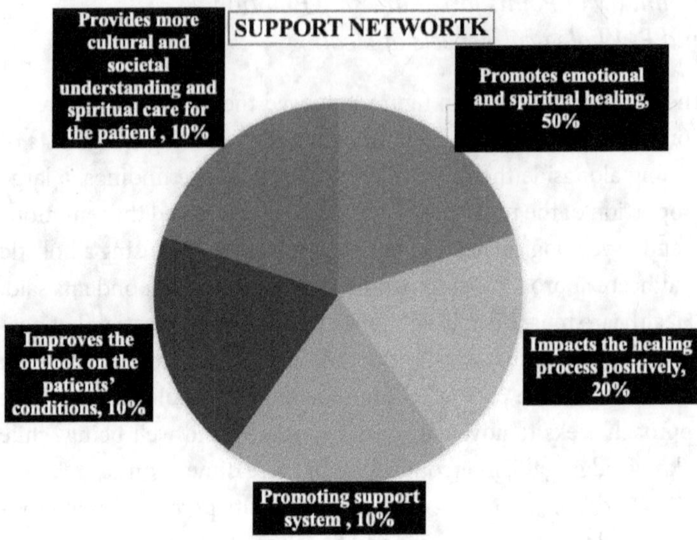

Figure 2. Support Network

Summary of Effectiveness of Support Networks in Promoting Spiritual and Emotional Healing for Cardiac Care Patients

The results presented in figure 2 show the respondents' perception on the effectiveness of support networks, such as those in the family and community, in promoting spiritual and emotional healing for cardiac care patients. The result revealed that 50 percent of the respondents perceived that support systems are effective in promoting emotional healing. One of the respondents said, "Every human being needs a support system. This could impact the healing process. A patient healing could be faster when the person feels connected to loved ones" (Respondent AB). Again, "the presence of the family and community, like the church, help promote spiritual and emotional healing in a way that they are the support group that provide strength and gives hope and uplift the spirit, especially when patient needs to undergo a major procedure like open heart" (Respondent EF). Another respondent said, "Family involvement in treatment can be utilized to help promote emotional healing. A strong family support system can help those with emotional trauma with resilience" (Respondent IJ). Going by the responses, support networks such as family, friends, loved ones, and community is perceived to be effective in promoting emotional healing of cardiac patients.

Support networks can be effective in impacting the healing process (20 percent). According to one of the respondents, "I think first, a person needs to have a good support system to be able to utilize them. If one is established, I myself find that this, most often than not, tends to happen on its own. A great support system almost always, in my opinion, is associated with a promotion of spiritual or emotional healing, regardless of the type of patient" (Respondent CD). In agreement with the result, a respondent said,

> Bringing support networks together is important. Things can seem overwhelming to a patient. Questions, worries, trouble navigating information can all be too much for one person to manage. A place to start within the hospital could possibly be a location designated to help begin emotional healing. I would describe it as an area someone could calm down without the "clinical" atmosphere. Support staff present could offer assistance or just some positive conversation for someone under the stress of illness. (Respondent MN)

Furthermore, the results showed that support networks are equally effective in improving the outlook on the patients' conditions, promoting the support systems, and providing more cultural and societal understanding and spiritual care for the patient.

Research Question 3

How can healthcare institutions create an environment that fosters collaboration and communication among multidisciplinary teams, including physicians, nurses, chaplains, social workers, and mental health professionals, to provide holistic healing for patients?

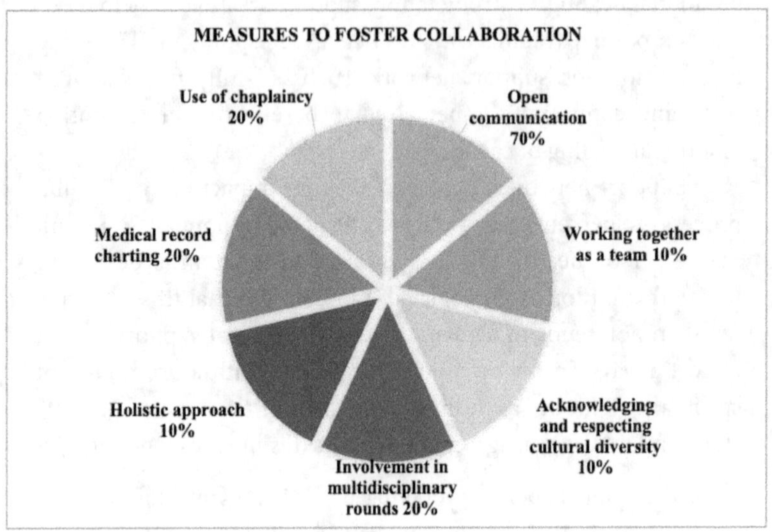

Figure 3. Measures to Foster Collaboration and Communication Among Multidisciplinary Teams

Summary of Measures to Foster Collaboration and Communication Among Multidisciplinary Teams in Providing Holistic Healing for Patients

Results for figure 3 revealed the respondents' perception on how healthcare institutions can create an environment that fosters collaboration and communication among multidisciplinary teams, including physicians, nurses, chaplains, social workers, and mental health professionals, to provide holistic healing for patients. According to the results, a majority of the respondents (70 percent) perceived that open communication among healthcare providers can help foster collaboration among them. This is plausible in that open communication can help healthcare providers to share ideas, compare notes, and understand the best possible approach to handle specific patients. Emphasizing the need for open communication, one respondent said,

> The healthcare institutions can create an environment that foster collaboration and communication among multidisciplinary teams, including physicians, nurses, chaplains, social workers and mental health professionals, to provide holistic healing for patients by delivering consistent care through daily rounds; assessment of physical, mental, emotional, spiritual, and social needs of patients and addressing their needs; providing important information about their test results and treatment; calling family for update of care and patient's condition; and most especially by acknowledging and respecting diversity of culture. (Respondent GH)

This can be achieved with open communication among healthcare providers. Another respondent emphatically stated that "healthcare professionals must work together to foster the total healing of the person. This process includes collaborations that is engaged with open communication" (Respondent EF).

The result also identified working as a team (20 percent) and being involved in multidisciplinary rounds (20 percent) and medical record charting (20 percent) as some of the measures with which healthcare institutions create an environment that fosters collaboration and communication among multidisciplinary teams, including physicians, nurses, chaplains, social workers, and mental health professionals, to provide holistic healing for patients. One of the respondents affirmed that "one aspect of fostering collaboration that I have found to have helped me is being involved in multidisciplinary rounds, where team members from various disciplines come together to discuss patient cases, share insights, and collaboratively develop care plans" (Respondent OP). The results strongly affirmed that collaboration can be fostered when the healthcare institutions create an environment for open communication, teamwork, and sharing of information among healthcare providers. It will equally improve a professional's effectiveness in providing holistic healing to one's patient.

Research Question 4

What are the existing barriers and factors that affect the integration of spiritual and emotional care into the cardiac care journey, both within healthcare institutions and among healthcare providers?

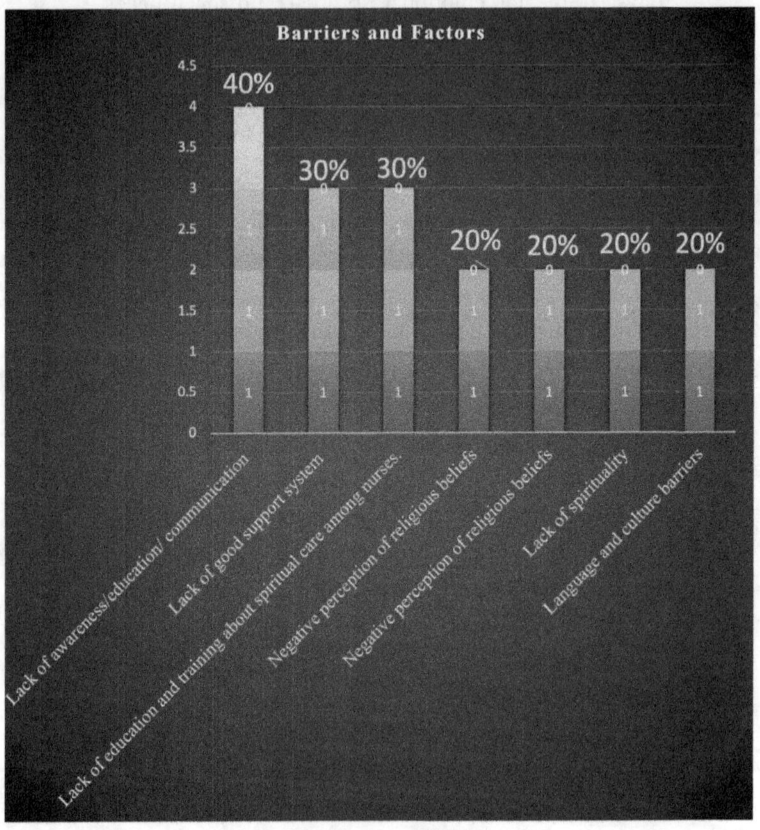

Figure 4. Barriers and Factors

Summary of Barriers and Factors that Affect the Integration of Spiritual and Emotional Care

Findings for figure 4 revealed the respondents' perceptions on the existing barriers and factors that affect the integration of spiritual and emotional care in the cardiac care journey, both within health-care institutions and among healthcare providers. The result revealed that some of the existing barriers were lack of awareness/education/communication (40 percent), lack of education and training about spiritual care among nurses (30 percent), lack of a good support system (30 percent), individual barriers like lack of interest in nursing (20 percent), negative perception of religious beliefs (20 percent), language and culture barriers (20 percent), and lack of spirituality, among others (see appendix D). This finding affirms that there are existing barriers and factors affecting the effective integration of spiritual and emotional care into the cardiac care journey, both within healthcare institutions and among healthcare providers. A respondent clearly asserts,

> Barriers is that, in a hospital setting, we work in a very diverse population where clinicians are often pressed to focus on the impersonal diagnosis of a disease and organ dysfunction. They do not have the tools, language, emotional energy, to explore the patient, who has come from their own livelihood, in other dimensions. Hence, clinicians may not have the time, language, or ability to facilitate, to go beyond the labs, disease, or body in front of them, into their former activity and social participation. They rely on the Case Management whose role is to expedite discharge. (Respondent AB)

Another respondent simply affirmed that "one easy answer is that some lack spirituality, leading to a lack of healing options considered. Another could be the lack of a good support system, who again, I believe drives more spiritual/emotional healing" (Respondent KL).

These barriers consequently affect the functionality and effectiveness of healthcare in addressing spiritual and emotional care of patients. As opined by one respondent, "limited understanding of spiritual care in healthcare, lack of education of the support chaplaincy can provide and religious prejudice against faith in a healthcare setting are some of the factors negatively influencing spiritual and emotional healing of patients" (Respondent MN).

These barriers must be addressed for effective health service delivery by healthcare providers.

Research Question 5

How can integration of spiritual and emotional care interventions into the Annual HealthStream Education impact patient's holistic healing process?

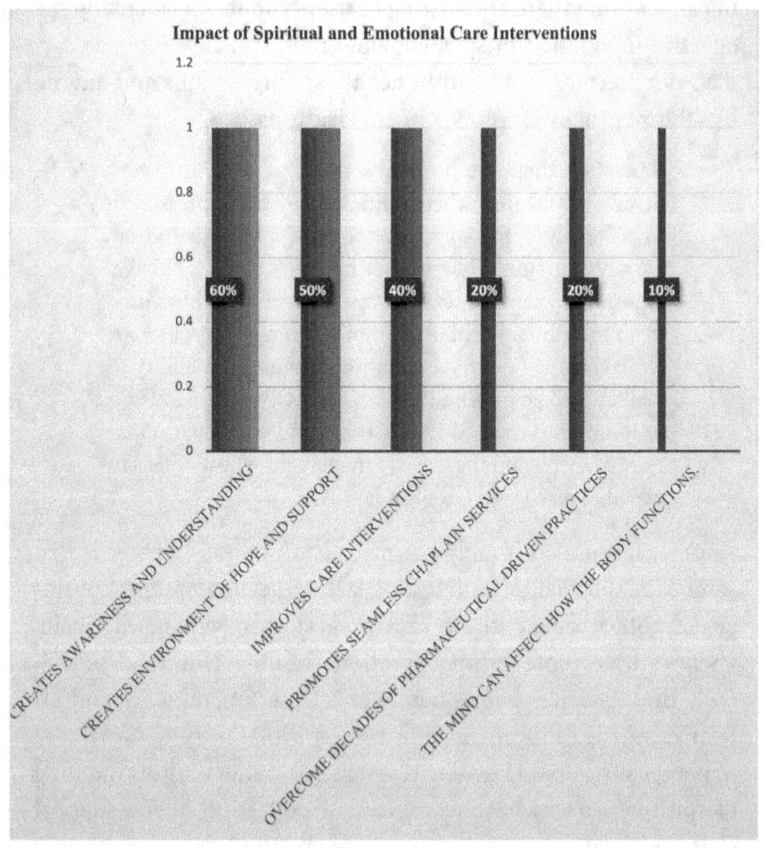

Figure 5. Impact of Spiritual and Emotional Care Interventions

*Summary of the Impact of Integration of Spiritual and
Emotional Care Interventions into the Annual HealthStream
Education on Patients' Holistic Healing Process*

The results for figure 5 show the perceptions of the respondents on the integration of spiritual and emotional care interventions in the annual HealthStream education program, focusing on the patient's holistic healing process. The results showed that 60 percent of the responses affirmed the integration of spiritual and emotional care interventions into the annual HealthStream education on patients' holistic healing process creates awareness and understanding of the need for spiritual and emotional care for patients (see appendix E). A respondent emphasized that "the spiritual and emotional aspects of a person must never be neglected during a care plan of patients. When bodily injury occurs in a patient, care providers must work along with other health care team members that would provide spiritual and emotional care" (Respondent EF). In line with the result, one respondent emphasized that

> integrating spiritual and emotional care interventions into a hospital's continuing education program, either in person or online, can help increase awareness and understanding of the spiritual and emotional factors that impact a person's overall health. It can help caregivers develop strategies for assessing these factors and then to learn strategies and techniques to assist themselves and their patients to address these aspects of healing. (Respondent KL)

The result showed that 50 percent of the responses suggested the integration of spiritual and emotional care interventions into the annual HealthStream education program on patient's holistic healing process creates awareness and understanding of the need for spiritual and emotional care for patients to create an environment of hope and support for the patients. This serves as huge emotional relief for the patients and boosts the healing process. A respondent posited that

> integrating spiritual and emotional care into Health-
> Stream education benefits the patient and the healthcare
> worker. I think it is important to," create an environment
> of hope and support. Recognizing physical needs within
> the healthcare setting is only one part of a patient's jour-
> ney. (Respondent GH)

Other impacts of the integrating spiritual and emotional care interventions into the annual HealthStream education for patients' holistic healing processes were to improve care interventions (40 percent), to overcome decades of pharmaceutical driven practices (20 percent), and promote seamless chaplain services (20 percent), among others (see appendix E).

SUMMARY OF RESULTS

The findings revealed a holistic healthcare approach is the best approach in addressing the spiritual and emotional healing process of cardiac patients. The finding is plausible in that a holistic approach seeks to advance general harmony and well-being while acknowledging the interconnection of these dimensions. Hvidt et al. asserts that spiritual care (SC), which is an aspect of holistic care, improves patients' quality of life, and the absence of SC is linked to existential and spiritual suffering, which can lead to a higher risk of depression and deteriorated health, leading to higher health-care expenses.[13] Holistic care recognizes a person as a whole and acknowledges the interdependence of the biological, social, psychological, and spiritual aspects. Corroborating with the findings, holistic healing takes the full person into account, addressing not only physical ailments but also an individual's emotional, mental, and spiritual needs. Roberts views holistic care as a treatment philosophy that sets dissimilar and high expectations for quality of care, both for healthcare facilities and for all the interdisciplinary team.[14] In holistic healthcare, all aspects of a patient's treatment process are considered and the patients' thoughts, emotions,

---

13. Hvidt et al., "What Is Spiritual Care?," 2.

14. Roberts, *Professional Spiritual and Pastoral Care*, 23.

cultures, opinions, and attitudes are factored in as contributing to recovery, happiness, and satisfaction.

The findings affirmed that support networks, such as those in the family and community, help in promoting spiritual and emotional healing for cardiac care patients. It is expected that a strong support system will promote emotional and spiritual healing. Even a self-centered person naturally wishes to have the kind of fiber willing to shoulder a fair portion of the agony and work because of this desire.[15] Support system and networks aid in providing emotional and spiritual support, such as active listening, understanding patient behavior during discomfort, offering words of comfort, and acknowledging cultural beliefs, cultivating positivity, relying on prayer, family, and friends. The findings strongly associated emotional and spiritual healing with effective support systems/networks in healthcare services. The presence of family and friends plays a great role in the healing process of a patient and, therefore, cannot be overemphasized. Thus, to feel dignified, one must be looked for by others.[16]

The findings affirmed that open communication among healthcare institutions creates an environment that fosters collaboration and communication among multidisciplinary teams, including physicians, nurses, chaplains, social workers, and mental health professionals, to provide holistic healing for patients. This is plausible in that open communication can help healthcare providers to share ideas, compare notes, and understand the best possible approach to handle specific patients. Effective communication helps to foster engagement, cooperation, and information sharing among multidisciplinary healthcare units and teams to ensure holistic healing of patients. Effective spiritual care requires strong communication skills to facilitate open, empathetic, and nonjudgmental conversations about patients' beliefs and values. It helps one to share what is in their mind and heart without fear of criticism, contempt, or defensiveness, barriers that could be detrimental to effective communication. A study showed that

15. Houselander, *Guilt*, 120.

16. Brooks, *Love Your Enemies*, 69.

discussing existential or spiritual issues with patients can lead to touchy subjects; however, good team communication and continuity of care needs to be balanced against the need for efficient collaboration and continuity of care.[17] To foster collaboration through effective communication, it is essential for healthcare personnel to receive training and ongoing education in communication techniques that are specifically tailored to fostering more effective and empathetic spiritual care.

The findings also confirmed that there were existing barriers and factors that affected the integration of spiritual and emotional care into the cardiac care journey, both within healthcare institutions and among healthcare providers. These barriers were lack of awareness/education/communication, lack of education and training about spiritual care among nurses and other healthcare professionals, lack of good support systems, individual barriers like lack of interest in nursing, negative perception of religious beliefs, language, culture barriers, and lack of spirituality, among others. Institutional factors, such as lack of a good support system, lack of clear institutional policies, high level of provider burnout, lack of time due to short staffing, and lack of continuity affected the integration of spiritual and emotional care. Some researchers point out that lack of time and money are some of the reasons given by professionals for not prioritizing SC.[18]

The findings equally affirmed the integration of spiritual and emotional care interventions into the annual HealthStream education on patients' holistic healing process creates awareness and understanding of the need for spiritual and emotional care for patients and creates an environment of hope and support for the patients. This result is consistent with the researcher's presumption that the inclusion of spiritual and emotional support interventions in the yearly HealthStream education program will greatly alleviate patients' emotional distress and enable their quick recovery. By teaching staff members about the theory of the underlying conduct that is deemed challenging and how to enhance one's work

17. Keall et al., "How Do Australian Palliative," 3202.

18. Hvidt et al., "What Is Spiritual Care?," 2.

practices, healthcare professionals can better meet the unique needs of their care recipient.[19] Creating a welcoming environment that accommodates diverse spiritual practices and provides access to chaplains, spiritual counselors, or support groups can enhance the integration of spirituality in healthcare. According to Roberts, safe spaces where a care receiver can freely share experiences under the supervision of a caregiver who addresses this sacred time with creativity, compassion, collaboration, and competence are necessary to support a person's quest for healing.[20] By doing so, healthcare providers can promote holistic well-being, emotional resilience, and improved patient outcomes while nurturing a sense of comfort, purpose, and connectedness for individuals facing health challenges.

19. Smith et al., "Qualitative Study," 577.
20. Roberts, *Professional Spiritual and Pastoral Care*, 122.

5

Conclusion

Based on the reviews in the previous chapters, and with the outcomes of the intervention implementation detailed in chapters 3 and 4, this concluding chapter aims to answer the "so what" question. A thorough examination has revealed that providing for the spiritual needs of hospitalized patients is a crucial but sometimes disregarded component of patient care.[1] The need to develop and implement a model of holistic healing for integrating spiritual and emotional care alongside physical treatment has been the focus of the author. This study dug deep into the worlds of pastoral care and its transformational influence on holistic healing, and the results and conclusion of this are reflected in a larger context of pastoral care practices in the healthcare industry.

This chapter critically analyzed the research implication, how the findings of this research work will be applied to the patient's transformative healing journey, limitations that research may encounter, and areas for further research. It clarifies the various ways in which spiritual care goes beyond the limits of traditional healthcare, promoting mental, spiritual, and psychosocial well-being, and shows how spiritual care practitioners help patients dealing with

---

1. Kirchoff et al., "Spiritual Care of Inpatients," 1419.

serious health issues find resilience and a feeling of completeness by acting as catalysts for transformative healing journeys.

This study also outlines a road map for healthcare organizations looking to improve health professionals' ability to offer complete, patient-centered care through an examination of best practices and potential development areas. The findings highlight the potential for interaction between the medical and spiritual facets of care and stress the demand for a more inclusive strategy that considers patients' various spiritual needs and beliefs. This chapter acts as a forum for meaningful discussion and a call to action, asking healthcare stakeholders to acknowledge the crucial role of spiritual care in fostering holistic healing and establishing a more compassionate and inclusive healthcare model.

RESEARCH IMPLICATIONS

In the field of healthcare, the importance of comprehending and treating the whole person, including the body and spirit, has come to be better understood. The need to create and implement a holistic healing model for cardiac care patients goes beyond specific patient outcomes to encompass more general facets of healthcare delivery, relationships between providers and patients, cost-effectiveness, and evidence-based practice. So, "holistic care" has become a widely accepted idea, and according to studies, a holistic approach to care improves patient happiness and efficiency.[2] By recognizing the interconnectedness of physical, spiritual, and emotional dimensions of health, this research has the potential to transform the way healthcare is conceptualized and delivered, ultimately leading to improved quality of care and better outcomes for patients with cardiovascular diseases. Below are some implications that emerged from the findings:

2. Roberts, *Professional Spiritual and Pastoral Care*, 23.

Holistic Care

When providing treatment and support, holistic care considers the needs of the patient, body, mind, and spirit. Holistic care acknowledges the interdependence of many facets of a person's well-being, in contrast to traditional medical paradigms that frequently focuses on the outward manifestations of an illness or condition. This method places a strong emphasis on the value of addressing lifestyle, environment, social support, and personal beliefs in addition to current health issues. Rather than focusing only on treating specific issues or controlling symptoms, healthcare professionals strive to promote overall well-being and healing by adopting a holistic approach. Respondent EF posits,

> As a CCU Nurse, I listen to patients' complaints and address their needs as they arise. I try to understand and accept their behavior as they are experiencing discomforts and provide the appropriate treatment they need. I also offer emotional support through spending time talking to them, and giving words of comfort acknowledging their culture and beliefs, and make referral for follow-ups where and when necessary.

In holistic care, "each individual has to be treated as a unique being with a unique kind of spirituality and with unique values associated to that spirituality."[3] Treatment plans are tailored to everyone's unique needs and circumstances, acknowledging that what works for one person may not work for another. This could entail a mix of traditional medical treatments, complementary therapies like acupuncture or meditation, food adjustments or exercise plans, lifestyle adjustments, and psychosocial support. The goal is to empower individuals to take an active role in one's own health and to address the underlying causes of illness or imbalance, rather than just alleviating surface-level symptoms. By viewing health through a holistic lens, healthcare providers can foster a deeper understanding of their patients' experiences and promote more comprehensive healing and well-being.

3. Hvidt et al., "What Is Spiritual Care?," 8.

The research implications from this theme suggest that healthcare providers, as a team, ought to pay attention to the spiritual and physical needs of patients, listen to patients' complaints, understand and accept everyone's behavior, and offer emotional support. There is also the need to cultivate a positive mindset, paying attention to the patient's needs, and providing physical, social, spiritual, and emotional support.

Support System

Implications from this research study assert that when it comes to spiritual care, a person's support system is essential in helping the person feel at ease, guided, and inspired as the patient travels through life. This network often includes religious leaders, community members, friends, family, and healthcare professionals who are sensitive to the spiritual needs of the individual. These people provide a secure environment for the expression and investigation of ideas, values, and existential issues.

According to the findings, the research implications from above revealed that 50 percent of the respondents perceived that support systems are effective in promoting emotional healing. Thus, one of the respondents said, "Every human being needs a support system. This could impact the healing process. A patient healing could be faster when the person feels connected to loved ones" (Respondent AB). Also, "the presence of the family and community, like the church, help promote spiritual and emotional healing in a way that they are the support group that provide strength and gives hope and uplift the spirit, especially when patient needs to undergo a major procedure like open heart" (Respondent EF).

Within this network, religious leaders and spiritual guides offer guidance rooted in faith traditions, providing rituals, prayers, and scriptures that offer solace and meaning. Patients who feel or experience unmet spiritual needs report being less satisfied with the overall care and quality of treatment received.[4] Also, "patients

4. O'Brien et al., "Meeting Patients' Spiritual Needs," 183.

with unmet spiritual needs are at increased risk of poorer psychological outcomes, diminished quality of life, reduced sense of spiritual peace and increased risk of depression."[5] Ironically, since spirituality is a basic aspect of who one is as a person, it demands that spiritual care be a well-integrated part of healthcare. However, this makes practicing spiritual care challenging, as each person must be recognized as an individual with a unique spirituality and set of values that go along with it.[6]

Furthermore, improved patient well-being is strongly correlated with a supportive hospital environment that places a high priority on patient-centered care. To do this, environments that make patients feel listened to, respected, and appreciated must be established. This will promote cooperation and confidence between patients and healthcare providers. In addition, treatment regimens that incorporate complementary therapies like music therapy, art therapy, and mindfulness practices help address the psychological and emotional components of health and promote overall well-being. Beyond the therapeutic context, social support networks and community involvement are also essential for sustaining patient wellness.

Effective Communication and Collaboration

This subtheme emphasizes how important it is to collaborate and communicate well to improve patient outcomes in a hospital setting. For communication to be effective, patients' spiritual and emotional needs must also be met in addition to medical knowledge. According to this research study, patients frequently want conversations about spiritual values and beliefs and to be a part of their healthcare experience. Therefore, to comprehend and handle these aspects of care, healthcare personnel must communicate in an open and sympathetic manner.

5. O'Brien et al., "Meeting Patients' Spiritual Needs," 183.
6. Hvidt et al., "What Is Spiritual Care?," 8.

According to the research findings in chapter 4, 70 percent of the respondents perceived open communication among healthcare providers can help foster collaboration among the interdisciplinary team and patient. This is plausible in that open communication can help healthcare providers to share ideas, compare notes, and understand the best possible approach to handle specific patient's needs. In a research study carried out by Keall, Clayton, and Butow, several nurses stated that providing spiritual care requires effective communication skills.[7]

Strengthening the bonds between patients and providers is essential to improving healthcare results and everyone's level of happiness. These connections are based on effective communication, which promotes cooperation, understanding, and trust. Patients feel appreciated and in control of their care when healthcare professionals actively listen to them, respect their viewpoints, and involve the patient in joint decision-making procedures. In accordance with the informed consent principle, caregivers must provide participants with all the details required in decision processes[8] and ensure that the individual's rights and welfare are protected.[9] Furthermore, open and honest communication about available treatments, possible side effects, and anticipated results boost self-assurance and ease fear, promoting better treatment compliance and better health results. Additionally, building rapport and empathy can assist medical professionals in comprehending the special requirements and worries of the patients, enabling the provision of more efficient and individualized care.

Therefore, this study's implications suggest the need for healthcare organizations to foster a collaborative environment, where interdisciplinary teams work together seamlessly to provide patient-centered care that encompasses spiritual dimensions. Also, it highlights the importance of effective communication and collaboration in enhancing patient care outcomes. By incorporating spiritual assessment and communication skills into healthcare

7. Keall et al., "How Do Australian Palliative," 3202.

8. Redman and Caplan, "Should the Regulation of Research," 38.

9. Abay et al., "Rapid Ethical Assessment," 12.

provider training and fostering interdisciplinary collaboration, healthcare organizations can better meet the spiritual needs of patients, improve patient's overall well-being, and promote a more holistic approach to healthcare delivery.

Education for Healthcare Interventions

Since healthcare systems are realizing more and more how vital it is to satisfy patients' spiritual and emotional needs in addition to one's physical health, it is imperative that spiritual and emotional care education be incorporated into healthcare professional education programs. Integrating such interventions into Swedish Hospital's annual HealthStream education program has significant research implications for enhancing patient-centered care and health outcomes. In many ways, attending to patients' needs for SC and spiritual reintegration calls for significant and diverse training of HCPs than providing physical, psychological, and social rehabilitation.[10]

With 60 percent of the responses affirming that the integration of spiritual and emotional care interventions into the annual HealthStream education on patients' holistic healing process creates awareness and understanding of the need for spiritual and emotional care for patients, it shows a positive implication. Thus, one of the respondents emphasized that

> integrating spiritual and emotional care interventions into a hospital's continuing education program either in person or online can help increase awareness and understanding of the spiritual and emotional factors that impact a person's overall health. It can help caregivers develop strategies for assessing these factors and then to learn strategies and techniques to assist themselves and their patients to address these aspects of healing. (Respondent MN)

10. Hvidt et al., "What Is Spiritual Care?," 8.

The findings suggest that integrating spiritual and emotional care interventions into healthcare education can lead to better patient satisfaction, reduced levels of anxiety and depression, and improved overall well-being. By incorporating modules on spiritual assessment, empathetic communication, and coping strategies for emotional distress, both Swedish and other hospitals' annual HealthStream education can empower healthcare professionals to provide more comprehensive care that addresses the holistic needs of patients. This training encourages staff to think about the individual's needs, through the teaching of theory behind behavior perceived as challenging, and ways in which healthcare professionals can improve their working practice.[11]

Furthermore, research indicates that healthcare providers who receive training in spiritual and emotional care interventions demonstrate increased confidence and competence in addressing these aspects of patient care. Integrating such content into the annual HealthStream education program can equip healthcare professionals with the knowledge and skills needed to effectively support patients facing spiritual and emotional challenges, fostering a therapeutic environment built on trust and compassion.

Research implications suggest integrating spiritual and emotional care interventions into healthcare education can contribute to a more resilient and engaged healthcare workforce while limiting burnout. According to a study, burnout is an overwhelming condition of emotional weariness, dehumanization of patients, and feelings of inadequacy on the part of the practitioner. It has a negative impact on providing compassionate treatment and productivity at work.[12] Thus, healthcare professionals who feel supported in addressing the spiritual and emotional needs of patients can experience lower levels of burnout and higher job satisfaction. By prioritizing the well-being of healthcare professionals through comprehensive education and support, health professionals can cultivate a culture of compassion and resilience that ultimately benefits patients and providers.

11. Smith et al., "Qualitative Study," 577.

12. Okoli et al., "Cross-Sectional Examination," 477.

Barriers and Factors Affecting Integration of Spiritual Care

The integration of spiritual care into healthcare settings is crucial for providing holistic and patient-centered care. However, several barriers and factors can affect the successful implementation of spiritual care interventions. Understanding these challenges is essential for developing strategies to overcome them and promote effective integration of spiritual care into healthcare practice.

One significant barrier to the integration of spiritual care is a lack of awareness or understanding among healthcare providers about the importance of addressing patients' spiritual needs. From the research, many healthcare professionals receive limited training in spiritual care during their education and may feel ill-equipped to broach spiritual topics with patients. Additionally, misconceptions or biases about spirituality and religion may hinder open communication and collaboration between healthcare providers and patients. A respondent affirmed that and stated, "One easy answer is that some lack spirituality" (Respondent GH).

From the data analysis, the results revealed that some of the existing barriers were lack of awareness/education/communication (40 percent), lack of training about spiritual care among nurses (30 percent), lack of good support systems (30 percent), individual barriers like lack of interest in nursing (20 percent), negative perception of religious beliefs (20 percent), language and cultural barriers (20 percent), and lack of spirituality, among others. More so, the literature reviewed has it that training medical staff by hospitals on spiritual care issues has positive effects on patients' well-being,[13] and inadequate training is the strongest predictor of rare spiritual care provision.[14] Additionally, institutional factors, such as time constraints and competing priorities, can hinder the integration of spiritual care into healthcare practice.

Cultural and religious diversity among patients also presents challenges to the integration of spiritual care. Healthcare providers must navigate varying beliefs, values, and practices related

13. van de Geer et al., "Multidisciplinary Training," 224.

14. Mitchell et al., "Developing a Medical School Curriculum," 728.

to spirituality and religion, which can influence patients' preferences for spiritual care interventions. Language barriers, cultural taboos, and differing attitudes towards healthcare may further complicate communication and collaboration between providers and patients. In all of this, this research work affirms the need to understand that spiritual caregiving is a professional practice of compassionate ministry most frequently done in secular institutions, seeking accommodation for all without the establishment of a specific religion.[15]

Despite these barriers, several factors can facilitate the integration of spiritual care into healthcare settings. Education and training programs that raise awareness about the importance of spiritual care and provide healthcare professionals with the necessary skills and knowledge can promote successful integration. Thus, to increase team members' ability to provide patients with the spiritual care that is required, training is badly needed.[16] Additionally, creating supportive institutional cultures that prioritize patient-centered care and providing resources for addressing patients' spiritual needs can foster a more conducive environment for integrating spiritual care into healthcare practice. With this, healthcare organizations may improve the delivery of holistic, patient-centered care that successfully attends to patients' spiritual needs by addressing these hurdles and fostering elements that allow integration.

RESEARCH APPLICATIONS

These research findings offer valuable insights that can be practically applied to enhance patient and staff care at Swedish Hospital in Chicago, and other hospitals. These findings are set to enhance the overall patient experience, improve health outcomes, and cultivate a supportive and nurturing environment for patients and staff. The findings applicable to this research work are as follows.

15. Ali et al., *Mantle of Mercy*, 42.
16. Kang et al., "Meaning-Centered Spiritual Care," 2.

Implement Standardized Spiritual Assessment Tools

Implement standardized spiritual assessment tools, like FACT, HOPE, SPIRIT, to systematically evaluate patients' spiritual needs and preferences during intake assessments allows healthcare providers to tailor care plans accordingly. FACT is a spiritual assessment tool designed to assess a patient's *faith* or belief system, patient's *active involvement*, patient's *comfort* or *concerns*, and *treatment* plans.[17] HOPE also is used to assess a patient's sources of *hope, organized religion, personal spirituality*, and *effects* on medical care.[18] SPIRIT is another tool for assessing patient's *spiritual belief system, personal spirituality, integration* with a spiritual community, *ritualized practices* or *restrictions, implications* for medical practice, and *terminal events planning*.[19] These assessment tools provide information for intervention planning. By implementing standardized assessment tools and training staff on effective communication techniques, hospitals can ensure that patients' spiritual beliefs, values, and preferences are adequately addressed within the context of patient care, leading to a holistic healing approach and patient satisfaction.

Promoting a Healing Environment

Promoting a healing environment in the hospital setting can have profound effects on patients and staff. Research suggests that elements such as natural light, soothing colors, artwork, story books, religious resources, comfort blankets, and access to green spaces can contribute to reduced stress, anxiety, and pain levels among patients. Similarly, providing spaces for relaxation, meditation, and reflection can support staff well-being and resilience, ultimately enhancing job satisfaction and performance. By integrating these principles of holistic healing into the design and management of

---

17. LaRocca-Pitts, "FACT," 25.
18. LaRocca-Pitts, "FACT," 28.
19. LaRocca-Pitts, "FACT," 29.

hospitals spaces, they can create environments that promote healing and foster a sense of peace and comfort for all.

Educational Training for Healthcare Providers

Providing ongoing education and training opportunities for staff is essential for staying updated on the latest research and best practices in spiritual care and holistic healing. By offering annual education, workshops, seminars, new staff orientation, and continuing education programs, hospitals equip healthcare providers with the knowledge, skills, and resources needed to effectively integrate spiritual care into patient interactions. This approach not only enhances staff competence and confidence in addressing patients' holistic needs but also fosters a culture of learning, innovation, and continuous improvement within the organization.

Fostering Interdisciplinary Collaboration

Fostering interdisciplinary collaboration among healthcare providers is essential for delivering comprehensive care that addresses patients' physical, emotional, and spiritual needs holistically. By bringing together physicians, nurses, therapists, chaplains, and other professionals, healthcare organizations can develop integrated care plans that consider the whole person and promote holistic well-being. Regular interdisciplinary team meetings, joint care planning sessions, unit rounds, team referrals, and opportunities for shared learning and skill-building can strengthen collaboration and communication among staff, leading to more coordinated and effective care delivery. Through these collaborative efforts, Swedish Hospital and other healthcare systems can maximize the impact of research findings on spiritual care and holistic healing, ultimately improving patient outcomes and enhancing the overall quality of care provided.

Offering Supportive Services

Establishing support services, such as chaplaincy programs, counseling services, and support groups, to provide emotional and spiritual support to patients/families and staff during times of illness, grief, or loss is important. This approach encompasses various forms of assistance tailored to individuals' requirements, ranging from checking in with individuals, emotional support, and counseling to logistical aid, such as transportation, parking garage tickets, a cup of coffee/tea, and other assistance. Offering support services not only enhances the overall well-being of the care recipient but also increases the integrity and reliability of research findings. Moreover, it underscores a commitment to ethical research practices by prioritizing the holistic welfare of individuals involved, thereby promoting inclusivity, equity, and, ultimately, advancing scientific inquiry for the betterment of society.

Evaluating Outcomes and Quality Improvement

Regularly assessing patient outcomes, satisfaction levels, and staff well-being to gauge the effectiveness of spiritual care and holistic healing interventions and applying feedback to drive continuous quality improvement efforts should be considered. This process encompasses rigorous evaluation and systematically analyzing findings and identifying areas for improvement. Commitment to quality improvement not only ensures the integrity and credibility of this application but also fosters innovation and adaptation in response to evolving challenges and opportunities. In addition to ensuring the validity and integrity of this application, a dedication to quality improvement encourages creativity and adaptability in the face of changing possibilities and difficulties.

Summarily, the practical application of the research findings above can significantly enhance patient and staff care in healthcare organizations. By incorporating spiritual assessment into patient intake procedures, creating healing environments within the hospitals setting, fostering interdisciplinary collaboration among healthcare providers, and providing ongoing education and training opportunities for staff, Swedish and other hospitals can create a more patient-centered, supportive, and nurturing care environment that promotes holistic well-being for patients/families and staff.

RESEARCH LIMITATIONS

While the research on developing and implementing a model of holistic healing for cardiac care patients at Swedish Hospital in Chicago holds promise for improving patient outcomes and well-being, it is essential to acknowledge some limitations that impacted the interpretation and generalizability of the findings. These limitations include the following.

Ethical Consideration

Ethical considerations pose a significant challenge for the researchers investigating spiritual care as an art of holistic healing intervention, particularly when healthcare professionals serve as participants in the study. One projected ethical concern involved ensuring the voluntary and informed consent of the participants. The researcher also prioritized transparent communication, provided comprehensive information about the study objectives, risks, and benefits, and affirmed participants' rights to withdraw from the study at any time without repercussions. Upholding the principles of autonomy and respect for participants' decisions was essential for maintaining ethical integrity throughout the research process. Similarly, safeguarding the confidentiality and privacy of the participants was paramount, while also protecting the participant's professional standing and personal beliefs.

Spiritual care is often a deeply personal and sensitive topic, and healthcare professionals may be hesitant to share their experiences or perspectives if they fear breaches of confidentiality. Therefore, the researcher implemented strong data protection measures, such as anonymization and secure storage of data, to minimize the risk of inadvertent disclosure and maintain the trust and confidence of participants. Additionally, the researcher considered the potential impact of the study on participants' well-being, particularly as it involves exploring sensitive topics related to spirituality and holistic healing practices. Prioritizing participants' welfare and mitigating potential risks through ethical review and oversight mechanisms were essential steps the researcher took to ensure the ethical conduct of this study.

Cultural and Contextual Factors

Like any healthcare facility, Swedish Hospital functions within a particular cultural and contextual framework influenced by its location, the demographics of its patients, and its organizational culture. The cultural diversity among the participants influenced the perceptions, beliefs, and practices of respondents regarding the research study, which posed some challenges as the researcher tried to capture the full spectrum of perspectives. Cultural differences in understanding spirituality, illness, and healing influenced the participants' responses as well as participants' willingness to engage with spiritual care interventions, as the researcher experienced during participants' recruitment.

Navigating cultural and contextual factors made the researcher adopt a nuanced and culturally sensitive approach in carrying out the investigation. Sensitivity to cultural diversity and contextual nuances was essential for accurately interpreting participants' responses and ensuring the validity and reliability of the study findings. The researcher engaged with healthcare professionals from diverse cultural backgrounds and disciplines, acknowledging and respecting the multiplicity of perspectives on spirituality and holistic healing. By addressing cultural and contextual factors as inherent limitations in this research study, the researcher fostered greater inclusivity and relevance in the exploration of spiritual care as an integral component of holistic healing.

Participant Bias

As a limitation of this study, the researcher observed the respondents' biases ranging from individual beliefs, their understanding of spirituality, and personal experience of the topic under review. For instance, healthcare professionals with strong religious affiliations or spiritual beliefs may approach the topic of spiritual care with a predisposition toward certain practices or interventions, potentially affecting the objectivity of their feedback. Similarly, individuals' prior experiences with holistic healing or spiritual practices may color their perceptions of the effectiveness or relevance of such interventions within the healthcare setting. By acknowledging and addressing participants' biases, the researcher enhanced the credibility and relevance of participants' investigation into spiritual care as an essential component of holistic healing by creating a supportive and nonjudgmental research environment that encouraged open and honest dialogue among participants, allowing for the exploration of diverse perspectives and experiences related to spiritual care.

Time Constraint

Acknowledging and addressing time constraints as a limitation is essential for this research work. The demanding nature of the medical profession, coupled with the bustling environment of Swedish Hospital, presented some challenges in scheduling and conducting research activities. Healthcare professionals often have tight schedules filled with patient care duties, administrative tasks, and professional development commitments, leaving limited time for participation in other endeavors. So, the unpredictable nature of healthcare settings necessitated some rescheduling of interviews or data collection sessions due to emergent patient needs or unforeseen circumstances, which, in a way, almost affected the researcher's timeline. In some situations, these time constraints can impede the thoroughness and depth of data collection, potentially limiting the researchers' ability to capture the nuanced perspectives and experiences of the participants. That notwithstanding, the researcher carefully navigated these time constraints by adopting some flexibility with time to accommodate participants' schedules, to maximize the efficiency of the research procedures, and to optimize the quality and depth of data obtained within the available time frame.

In conclusion, even though the research on developing and implementing a model of holistic healing for cardiac care patients offers valuable insights into the potential benefits of integrating spiritual and emotional care alongside physical treatment, this subtheme recognized the importance of addressing these limitations, which could have affected the validity and reliability of this study. To optimize holistic care approaches that effectively meet the different needs of cardiac care patients, healthcare practitioners ought to acknowledge these limitations and incorporate them into future research and practice efforts.

FURTHER RESEARCH

As a recommendation for further investigation, exploring the impact of integrating spiritual care into various hospitals' annual HealthStream education, alongside other ongoing spiritual care education for the interdisciplinary team, holds significant promise. Understanding how such integration influences healthcare professionals' attitudes, knowledge, and practices regarding spiritual care can provide valuable insights into improving patient-centered care and addressing holistic patient needs. By conducting longitudinal studies or randomized controlled trials, the researcher can assess the effectiveness of these educational interventions in enhancing patient outcomes, satisfaction levels, and overall quality of care. Additionally, investigating potential barriers, facilitators, and best practices for integrating spiritual care education into existing training programs can inform the development of comprehensive, evidence-based approaches to spiritual care delivery within healthcare settings.

Appendix A

Participants' Demographics

S/N	Participants	Age	Profession	Experience
1	AB	36	Registered Nurse	5 years
2	CD	35	Registered Nurse	7.5 years
3	EF	50	Case Manager	25 years
4	GH	62	Physician	30 years and above
5	IJ	39	Physician	8 years
6	KL	53	Secretary/Unit Nurse Aid	17 years
7	MN	64	Registered Nurse	33 years
8	OP	75	Chaplain	22 years
9	QR	50	Registered Nurse	13 years

Appendix B

Interview Time Frame

Serial No.	Participants	Interview Time Frame
1	AB	25 minutes (11:00 a.m. to 11:25 a.m.)
2	CD	20 minutes (8:45 a.m. to 9:05 a.m.)
3	EF	17 minutes (12:30 p.m. to 12:47 p.m.)
4	GH	28 minutes (2:00 p.m. to 2:28 p.m.)
5	IJ	22 minutes (8:00 a.m. to 8:22 p.m.)
6	KL	31 minutes (4:00 p.m. to 4:31 p.m.)
7	MN	18 minutes (2:30 p.m. to 12:48 p.m.)
8	OP	32 minutes (4:20 p.m. to 4:52 p.m.)
9	QR	25 minutes (11:30 a.m. to 11:55 a.m.)

Appendix C

Summary of Points for Addressing Emotional and Psychological Aspects of Healing

S/N	Coded Responses	Response Frequency	%
1	Holistic healthcare approach	4	40.00
2	Collaboration	1	10.00
3	Communication	1	10.00
4	Positive mindset towards patients	1	10.00
5	Participatory approach	2	20.00
6	Goal setting	1	10.00
7	Prayers	1	10.00
8	Paying attention to the patient	1	10.00
9	Use of family and friends	3	30.00
11	Discussion with the patient	1	10.00

Note. Multiple responses recorded.

Appendix D

Summary of Points for Effectiveness of Support Networks in Promoting Spiritual and Emotional Healing for Cardiac Care Patients

S/N	Coded Responses	Response Frequency	%
1	Impacts the healing process positively	2	20.00
2	Promotes support system	1	10.00
3	Promotes emotional healing	5	50.00
4	Improves the outlook on the patients' conditions	1	10.00
5	Provides more cultural and societal understanding and spiritual care for the patient	1	10.00

Note. Multiple responses recorded.

Appendix E

Summary of Measures to Foster Collaboration and Communication Among Multidisciplinary Teams in Providing Holistic Healing for Patients

S/N	Coded Responses	Response Frequency	%
1	Open communication	7	70.00
2	Working together as a team	2	20.00
3	Acknowledging and respecting cultural diversity	1	10.00
4	Involvement in multidisciplinary rounds	2	20.00
5	Holistic approach	1	10.00
6	Medical record charting	2	20.00
7	Use of chaplaincy	1	10.00

Note. Multiple responses recorded.

Appendix F

Summary of Barriers and Factors that Affect the Integration of Spiritual and Emotional Care

S/N	Coded Responses	Response Frequency (n=9)	%
1	Neglect of some aspect of the care of the patient	1	10.00
2	Lack of continuity	1	10.00
3	Lack of education and training about spiritual care among nurses	3	30.00
4	Lack of time due to short staffing	1	10.00
5	Individual barriers, like lack of interest in nursing	2	20.00
6	Negative perception of religious beliefs	2	20.00
7	Problems in nurses' family relationship and financial problems	1	10.00
8	High level of provider burnout	1	10.00
9	Lack of clear institutional policies	1	10.00
10	Patients' varying comfort levels	1	10.00
11	Lack of spirituality	2	20.00

S/N	Coded Responses	Response Frequency (n=9)	%
12	Lack of good support system	3	30.00
13	Language and culture barriers	2	20.00
14	Lack of awareness/education/communication	4	40.00

Note. Multiple responses recorded.

Appendix G

Summary of the Impact of Integration of Spiritual and Emotional Care Interventions into the Annual HealthStream Education on Patients' Holistic Healing Process

S/N	Coded Responses	Response Frequency	%
1	The mind can affect how the body functions	1	10.00
2	It creates awareness and understanding of the need for spiritual care	6	60.00
3	It will improve care interventions	4	40.00
4	It can overcome decades of pharmaceutical driven practices	2	20.00
5	It creates an environment of hope and support	5	50.00
6	It promotes seamless chaplain services	2	20.00

Note. Multiple responses recorded.

Bibliography

Abay, Serebe, et al. "Rapid Ethical Assessment on Informed Consent Content and Procedure in Hintalo-Wajirat, Northern Ethiopia: A Qualitative Study." *PLoS ONE* 11.6 (2016) e0157056. https://doi.org/10.1371/journal.pone.0157056.

Abdolkarimi, Mahdi, et al. "The Relationship Between Spiritual Health and Happiness in Medical Students During the COVID-19 Outbreak: A Survey in Southeastern Iran." *Frontiers in Psychology* 13 (Aug. 2022) 974697. https://doi.org/10.3389/fpsyg.2022.974697.

Abu-El-Noor, Mysoon Khalil, and Nasser Ibrahim Abu-El-Noor. "Mapping the Road for a New Spiritual Care Policy: Identifying Barriers and Enhancing Factors for Providing Spiritual Care to Cardiac Patients." *Journal of Religion, Spirituality & Aging* 28.3 (2016) 184–99. https://doi.org/10.108 0/15528030.2015.1085482.

Adams, Michael, trans. *Major Prophets: Isaiah, Jeremiah, Ezekiel, Daniel.* The Navarre Bible: Text and Commentaries. Strongsville, OH: Scepter, 2005.

Ali, Muhammad A., et al., eds. *Mantle of Mercy: Islamic Chaplaincy in North America.* West Conshohocken, PA: Templeton, 2022.

Anim, Michael T., et al. "African Cultural Values in the Biopsychosocial-Spiritual Care Model to Manage Psychological Symptoms in Adults with Sickle Cell Disease in Ghana, West Africa." *Mental Health, Religion & Culture* 25.2 (2022) 177–96. https://doi.org/10.1080/13674676.2021.2025351.

Arrigo, Bruce, et al. "New Qualitative Methods and Critical Research Directions in Crime, Law, and Justice: Editors' Introduction." *Journal of Criminal Justice Education* 32.2 (2022) 145–50. https://doi.org/10.1080/10511253. 2022.2027484.

Baldwin, Jennifer. *Trauma-Sensitive Theology: Thinking Theologically in the Era of Trauma.* Eugene, OR: Cascade, 2018.

Best, Megan C., et al. "Australian Patient Preferences for the Introduction of Spirituality into Their Healthcare Journey: A Mixed Methods Study." *Journal of Religion and Health* 62 (Aug. 2022) 2323–40. https://doi. org/10.1007/s10943-022-01616-3.

Billups, Felice D. *Qualitative Data Collection Tools: Design, Development, and Applications.* Qualitiative Research Methods 55. Thousand Oaks, CA: Sage, 2021.

Brinkman-Stoppelenburg, Arianne, et al. "Involvement of Supportive Care Professionals in Patient Care in the Last Month of Life." *Supportive Care in Cancer* 23.10 (2015) 2899–906. https://doi.org/10.1007/s00520-015-2655-3.

Brooks, Arthur C. *Love Your Enemies: How Decent People Can Save America from the Culture of Contempt.* New York: HarperCollins, 2019.

Busetto, Loraine, et al. "How to Use and Assess Qualitative Research Methods." *Neurological Research and Practice* 2.14 (2020). https://doi.org/10.1186/s42466-020-00059-z.

Butler, Sarah A. *Caring Ministry: A Contemplative Approach to Pastoral Care.* New York: Continuum, 1999.

Cabral, Christie, et al. "Challenges to Implementing Electronic Trial Data Collection in Primary Care: A Qualitative Study." *BMC Family Practice* 22.147 (July 2021). https://doi.org/10.1186/s12875-021-01498-6.

Caecilie, B. Myrhoj, et al. "Interdisciplinary Collaboration in Serious Illness Conversations in Patients with Multiple Myeloma and Caregivers: A Qualitative Study." *BMC Palliative Care* 22.93 (2023). https://doi.org/10.1186/s12904-023-01221-5.

Casciaro, Jose Maria, ed. *St. John.* 2nd ed. Translated by Brian McCarthy. The Navarre Bible: Text and Commentaries. Dublin: Four Courts, 2005.

Clyne, Barbara, et al. "Patients' Spirituality Perspectives at the End of Life: A Qualitative Evidence Synthesis." *BMJ Supportive & Palliative Care,* 12.e4 (2019) e550–e561. https://doi.org/10.1136/bmjspcare-2019-002016.

Collins, Nina L. "The Jewish Source of Romans 5:17, 16, 10 and 9: The Verses of Paul in Relation to a Comment in the Mishnah at M. Makk 3.15." *Revue Biblique* 112.1 (2005) 27–45. https://www.jstor.org/stable/44090802.

Connolly, Greg, and Liza Oates. "The Wellness Industry: The Marginalization of Naturopathy and Western Herbal Medicine." *Australian Journal of Herbal and Naturopathic Medicine* 34.3 (2022) 102–8. https://www.researchgate.net/publication/363656087_The_wellness_industry_the_marginalisation_of_naturopathy_and_western_herbal_medicine.

Devers, Kelly, and Richard Frankel. "Study Design in Qualitative Research: Sampling and Data Collection Strategies." *Education for Health* 13.2 (2000) 263–71.

Duronjic, Andrea, et al. "The Impact of Language Barriers and Interpreters on Critical Care Patient Outcomes" *Journal of Critical Care* 73 (2023) 154182. https://doi.org/10.1016/j.jcrc.2022.154182.

Dutra, Claunei C. D., and Henrique S. Rocha. "Religious Support as a Contribution to Face the Effects of Social Isolation in Mental Health During the Pandemic of COVID-19." *Journal of Religious and Health* 60.1 (2021) 99–111. https://pubmed.ncbi.nlm.nih.gov/33405093/.

Er, Seda, et al. "The Effect of Psychosocial Distress and Self-Transcendence on Resilience in Patients with Cancer." *Perspectives in Psychiatric Care* 58.4 (2022) 2631–38. https://doi.org/10.1111/ppc.13103.

Finn, Laura, and Alva R. Roche. *Supportive Care Strategies: Optimizing Transplant Care.* Cham, Switzerland: Springer, 2020.

Fitchett, George. *Assessing Spiritual Needs: A Guide for Caregivers.* Lima, OH: Academic Renewal, 2002.

Garten, Lars, et al. "Palliative Care and Grief Counseling in Peri- and Neonatology: Recommendations from the German PaluTiN Group." *Frontiers in Pediatrics* 8.67 (2020). https://doi.org/10.3389/fped.2020.00067.

Gaudet, Stéphanie, and Dominique Robert. *A Journey Through Qualitative Research: From Design to Reporting.* Los Angelos: Sage, 2018. https://doi.org/10.4135/9781529716733.

George, Anne, et al. *Holistic Healthcare: Possibilities and Challenges.* Waretown, NJ: Apple, 2017.

Gibbs, Graham R. *Analyzing Qualitative Data.* London: Sage, 2018.

Gilliat-Ray, Sophie, et al. *Understanding Muslim Chaplaincy.* London: Routledge, 2016.

Grun, Anselm. *Jesus, the Image of Humanity: Luke's Account.* New York: Continuum, 2006.

Gustafson, Debra. *Departure Dialogues: Praying Like Jesus Prayed as He Faced Death.* Nashville: Missional, 2021.

Healy, Mary. *The Gospel of Mark: Catholic Commentary on Sacred Scripture.* Grand Rapids: Baker, 2008.

Henderson, Katherine, et al. "Patient Religiosity and Desire for Chaplain Services in an Outpatient Primary Care Clinic." *Journal of Pastoral Care & Counseling* 77 (2023) 81–89. https://pubmed.ncbi.nlm.nih.gov/36660791/.

Hills, Laura. "Overcoming the Ten Most Common Barriers to Effective Team Communication." *Journal of Medical Practice Management* 29.2 (2013) 99–103.

Houselander, Caryll. *Guilt.* Manchester, NH: Sophia, 2022.

Hvidt, Niels Christian, et al. "What Is Spiritual Care? Professional Perspectives on the Concept of Spiritual Care Identified Through Group Concept Mapping." *BMJ Open* 10.12 (2020) e042142. https://pubmed.ncbi.nlm.nih.gov/33372078/.

Jibiliza, Xolisa. "The Evolution of Pastoral Care Ministry through the Ages." *Pharos Journal of Theology* 102 (2021) 1–14. https://doi.org/10.46222/pharosjot.10211.

Jones, Andre L., et al. "The Spiritual Assessment." *Journal of American Family Physician* 106.4 (2022) 415–19. https://pubmed.ncbi.nlm.nih.gov/36260898/.

Joranger, Line. *An Interdisciplinary Approach to the Human Mind: Subjectivity, Science, and Experiences in Change.* Abingdon, UK: Routledge, 2019.

Kang, Kyung-Ah, et al. "A Meaning-Centered Spiritual Care Training Program for Hospice Palliative Care Teams in South Korea: Development and Preliminary Evaluation." *BMC Palliative Care* 20.1 (2021) 30. https://pubmed.ncbi.nlm.nih.gov/33563253/.

Keall, Robyn, et al. "How Do Australian Palliative Care Nurses Address Existential and Spiritual Concerns? Facilitators, Barriers, and Strategies." *Journal of Clinical Nursing* 23.21–22 (2014) 3197–205. https://doi.org/10.1111/jocn.12566.

Kelly, Ewan, and John Swinton, eds. *Chaplaincy and the Soul of Health and Social Care: Fostering Spiritual Wellbeing in Emerging Paradigms of Care.* London, Jessica Kingsley, 2019.

Kestenbaum, Allison, et al. "Spiritual AIM: Assessment and Documentation of Spiritual Needs in Patients with Cancer." *Journal of Health Care Chaplaincy* 28.4 (2021) 566–77. https://doi.org/10.1080/08854726.2021.2008170.

Kirchoff, Robert W., et al. "Spiritual Care of Inpatients Focusing on Outcomes and the Role of Chaplaincy Services: A Systematic Review." Journal of Religion and Health 6.2 (2021) 1406–22. https://doi.org/10.1007/s10943-021-01191-z.

Klimasinski, Maciej W. "Spiritual Care in the Intensive Care Unit." *Anesthesiology Intensive Therapy* 53.4 (2021) 350–57. https://pmc.ncbi.nlm.nih.gov/articles/PMC10165982/.

LaRocca-Pitts, Mark. "FACT, a Chaplain's Tool for Assessing Spiritual Needs in an Acute Care Setting." *Chaplaincy Today* 28.1 (2012) 25–32. https://www.tandfonline.com/doi/abs/10.1080/10999183.2012.10767446.

Lin, Xiaobiao, et al. "Exploring the Trend in Religious Diversity: Based on the Geographical Perspective." *PLoS ONE* 17.7 (2022) e0271343. https://doi.org/10.1371/journal.pone.0271343.

Lydon-Lam, Jennifer. "Models of Spirituality and Consideration of Spiritual Assessment." *International Journal of Childbirth Education* 27.1 (2012) 18–22. https://link.gale.com/apps/doc/A302298435/HRCA?u=anon~5e8faffa&sid=googleScholar&xid=38add106.

Macrae, Janet. Nightingale's Spiritual Philosophy and Its Significance for Modern Nursing. *Journal of Nursing Scholarship* 27.1 (1995) 8–10. https://doi.org/10.1111/j.1547-5069.1995.tb00806.x.

Magezi, Vhumani. "Positioning Care as 'Being with the Other' Within a Cross-Cultural Context: Opportunities and Challenges of Pastoral Care Provision Amongst People from Diverse Cultures." *Verbum et Ecclesia* 41.1 (2020) a2041. http://dx.doi.org/10.4102/ve.v41i1.2041.

Martelli, Sarah B. *Memory Eternal: Living with Grief as Orthodox Christians.* Chesterton, IN: Ancient Faith, 2022.

Mayeda, Donna P., and Katherine T. Ward. "Methods for Overcoming Barriers in Palliative Care for Ethnic/Racial Minorities: A Systematic Review." *Palliative and Supportive Care* 17.6 (2019) 697–706. https://doi.org/10.1017/s1478951519000403.

Mitchell, Christine M., et al. "Developing a Medical School Curriculum for Psychological, Moral, and Spiritual Wellness: Student and Faculty Perspectives." *Journal of Pain and Symptom Management* 52.5 (2016) 727–36. https://doi.org/10.1016/j.jpainsymman.2016.05.018.

Moitinho, Elias, and Denise Moitinho. *Dream Home: How to Create an Intimate Christian Marriage.* Dubuque, IA: Kendall Hunt, 2020.

Nacak, Ulviye Aydan, and Yasemin Erden. "End-of-Life Care and Nurse's Roles." *The Eurasian Journal of Medicine* 54.1 (2023) S141–44. https://doi.org/10.5152/eurasianjmed.2022.22324.

O'Brien, Mary R., et al. "Meeting Patients' Spiritual Needs During End-Of-Life Care: A Qualitative Study of Nurses' and Healthcare Professionals' Perceptions of Spiritual Care Training." *Journal of Clinical Nursing* 28.1–2 (2018) 182–89. https://doi.org/10.1111/jocn.14648.

Okoli, Chizimuzo T. C., et al. "A Cross-Sectional Examination of Factors Associated with Compassion Satisfaction and Compassion Fatigue Across Healthcare Workers in an Academic Medical Centre." *International Journal of Mental Health Nursing* 29.3 (2019) 476–87. https://doi.org/10.1111/inm.12682.

Olivi, Pierre Jean. "Commentary on the Gospel of Mark." Translated by Robert J. Karris. St. Bonaventure, NY: Franciscan Institute, 2011.

Ovadje, Lauretta, and Jerome Nriagu. "Multi-Dimensional Knowledge of Malaria Among Nigerian Caregivers: Implications for Insecticide-Treated Net Use by Children." *Malaria Journal* 15.1 (2016) 516. https://pubmed.ncbi.nlm.nih.gov/27769249/.

Peng-Keller, Simon, and David Neuhold. *Charting Spiritual Care: The Emerging Role of Chaplaincy Records in Global Health Care.* Cham, Switzerland: Springer Nature, 2020.

Pink, Arthur W. *Exposition of Hebrews.* Unabridged. Blacksburg, PA: Wilder, 2018.

Purabdollah, Majid, et al. "Intercultural Sensitivity, Intercultural Competence, and Their Relationship with Perceived Stress Among Nurses: Evidence from Iran." *Mental Health, Religion & Culture* 24.7 (2021) 687–97. https://doi.org/10.1080/13674676.2020.1816944.

Redman, Barbara K., and Arthur L. Caplan. "Should the Regulation of Research Misconduct Be Integrated with the Ethics Framework Promulgated in the Belmont Report?" *Ethics & Human Research* 43.1 (2021) 37–41. https://doi.org/10.1002/eahr.500078.

Reeve, Lucy, and Joanna Lavery. "Navigating Cultural Competence in District Nursing." *British Journal of Community Nursing* 28.7 (2023) 338–43. https://doi.org/10.12968/bjcn.2023.28.7.338.

Rehder, Kyle, et al. "The Science of Health Care Worker Burnout: Assessing and Improving Health Care Worker Well-Being." *Archives of Pathology & Laboratory Medicine* 145.9 (2021) 1095–109. https://pubmed.ncbi.nlm.nih.gov/34459858/.

Bibliography

Richardson, Ronald W. *Becoming a Healthier Pastor: Family Systems Theory and the Pastor's Own Family*. Minneapolis: Fortress, 2005.

Roberts, Stephen B. *Professional Spiritual and Pastoral Care: A Practical Clergy and Chaplain's Handbook*. 5th ed. Woodstock, VT: Skylight Paths, 2016.

Ryan, Robin. *God and the Mystery of Human Suffering: A Theological Conversation Across the Ages*. Mahwah, NJ: Paulist, 2011.

Schuhmann, Carmen, and Annelieke Damen. "Representing the Good: Pastoral Care in a Secular Age." *Journal of Pastoral Psychology* 67 (June 2018) 405–17. https://link.springer.com/article/10.1007/s11089-018-0826-0.

Sensing, Tim. *Qualitative Research: A Multi-Methods Approach to Projects for Doctor of Ministry Theses*. Eugene, OR: Wipf & Stock, 2011.

Smith, Raymond, et al. "A Qualitative Study Exploring Therapists' Experiences of Implementing a Complex Intervention Promoting Meaningful Activity for Residents in Care Homes." *Clinical Rehabilitation* 33.3 (2018) 575–83. https://doi.org/10.1177/0269215518815233.

Spatz, Erica S., et al. "The New Era of Informed Consent." *Journals of the American Medical Association* 315.19 (2016) 2063–64. https://doi.org/10.1001/jama.2016.3070.

Speyer, Cedric, and John Yaphe. *Applications of a Psychospiritual Model in the Helping Professions*. New York: Routledge, 2020.

Sprik, Petra J., et al. "Chaplains and Telechaplaincy: Best Practices, Strengths, Weaknesses—A National Study." *Journal of Health Care Chaplaincy* 29.1 (2022) 41–63. https://doi.org/10.1080/08854726.2022.2026103.

Sulmasy, Daniel P. "A Biopsychosocial-Spiritual Model for the Care of Patients at the End of Life." *Gerontologist* 42.3 (2002) 24–33. https://pubmed.ncbi.nlm.nih.gov/12415130/.

Summers, Charles A. "Matthew 14:13–21." *Interpretation: A Journal of Bible & Theology* 59.3 (2005) 298–99. https://journals.sagepub.com/doi/10.1177/002096430505900308.

Swedish Hospital, Part of NorthShore. *Department of Pastoral Care Orientation Manual*. Chicago: Swedish Hospital, 2023.

Swinton, John. *Finding Jesus in the Storm: The Spiritual Lives of Christians with Mental Health Challenges*. Grand Rapids: Eerdmans, 2020.

Tjale, Adele Agatha, and J. Bruce. "A Concept Analysis of Holistic Nursing Care in Paediatric Nursing." *Curationis* 30.4 (2007) 45–52. https://pubmed.ncbi.nlm.nih.gov/18402420/.

Tsosie, Krystal S., et al. "Considering 'Respect for Sovereignty' Beyond the Belmont Report and the Common Rule: Ethical and Legal Implications for American Indian and Alaska Native Peoples." *American Journal of Bioethics* 21.10 (2021) 27–30. https://doi.org/10.1080/15265161.2021.1968068.

Uytanlet, Samson L., and Kiem-Kiok Kwa. *Matthew: A Pastoral and Contextual Commentary*. Asia Bible Commentary Series. Carlisle: Langham, 2017.

van de Geer, Joep, et al. "Training Hospital Staff on Spiritual Care in Palliative Care Influences Patient-Reported Outcomes: Results of a Quasi-Experimental Study." *Palliative Medicine* 31.8 (2016) 743–53. https://doi.org/10.1177/0269216316676648.

Vermette, David, and Benjamin Doolittle. "What Educators Can Learn from the Biopsychosocial-Spiritual Model of Patient Care: Time for Holistic Medical Education." *Journal of General Internal Medicine* 37.8 (2022) 2062–66. https://pubmed.ncbi.nlm.nih.gov/35357678/.

Wolde, Ellen van. "Separation and Creation in Genesis 1 and Psalm 104, a Continuation of the Discussion of the Verb ברא." *Vetus Testamentum* 67.4 (2017) 611–47. https://www.jstor.org/stable/pdf/26566767.pdf?refreqid= excelsior%3Acef47adcd11e65fc56b8f6bb362ca513&ab_segments=&origi n=&initiator=&acceptTC=1.

Yang, Grace Meijuan, et al. "Effect of a Spiritual Care Training Program for Staff on Patient Outcomes." *Palliative and Supportive Care* 15.4 (2016) 434–43. https://doi.org/10.1017/s1478951516000894.

Yi-Chien, Chiang, et al. "A Spiritual Education Course to Enhance Nursing Students' Spiritual Competencies." *Nurse Education in Practice* 49 (Nov. 2020) 102907. https://doi.org/10.1016/j.nepr.2020.102907.

Zylla, Phil C. *The Roots of Sorrow: A Pastoral Theology of Suffering.* Waco, TX: Baylor University Press, 2012.